# YOUR CHILD
# IN THE
# HOSPITAL

*A Practical Guide for Parents*

# YOUR CHILD IN THE HOSPITAL

*A Practical Guide for Parents*

Second Edition

Nancy Keene & Rachel Prentice

O'REILLY®

Beijing • Cambridge • Köln • Paris • Sebastopol • Taipei • Tokyo

*Your Child in the Hospital: A Practical Guide for Parents, Second Edition*
by Nancy Keene and Rachel Prentice

Copyright © 1999, 1997 O'Reilly & Associates, Inc. All rights reserved.
Printed in the United States of America.

Published by O'Reilly & Associates, Inc., 101 Morris Street, Sebastopol,
CA 95472.

*Editor:* Linda Lamb
*Project Manager:* Claire Cloutier LeBlanc
*Production Services:* Kathleen Wilson

*Printing History:*

| | |
|---|---|
| October 1997: | First Edition |
| March 1999: | Second Edition |

*Library of Congress Cataloging-in-Publication Data*
Keene, Nancy.
    Your child in the hospital : a practical guide for parents / Nancy Keene & Rachel
      Prentice.—2nd ed.
      p. cm.—(Patient-centered guides)
    Includes bibliographical references.
    ISBN 1-56592-573-4 (pbk.)
    1. Children—Hospital care. 2. Sick children—Psychology. 3. Parent and child.
I. Prentice, Rachel. II. Title. III. Series.
RJ242 .K44 1999
362.1'1'083—dc21

                                          99-19134
                                            CIP

# Table of Contents

# Introduction

WHY DO I HAVE TO GO TO THE HOSPITAL? Will they hurt me? Are you going to leave me there? How long will I stay? These are some of the questions your child might ask before a trip to the hospital. Hospitals are fascinating, but sometimes frightening, places for children. They are full of beds with bars, buzzing machinery, and unfamiliar adults. Your child may be sick or hurt when she first enters this strange, new place. She may also be very worried.

For a parent, taking a child to the hospital can be scary as well. You must put your child in someone else's hands and you may think that there is no way to ease your child's fears. Actually, you can do plenty to prepare your child both physically and emotionally. You can learn about your child's illness or injury and answer her questions honestly. You can help your child feel safe and comfortable. You can work in partnership with the medical team to give your child the very best that medicine has to offer. And, as "extra eyes and ears" in the hospital, you can help prevent mistakes.

Knowing what the hospital is like can make it a lot easier to go there. That's what this book is for: to help you and your child prepare for and cope with the hospital experience. Over forty parents share stories about their own children's hospitalizations and offer advice based on their experiences. They tell how they answered their children's questions, cleared up misconceptions, and got them ready to go. Their stories show how good preparation transformed many of their children's fears into curiosity and cooperation.

These hospital veterans will also help you know what to expect once you and your child get to the hospital. They share methods to make hospital routines predictable, and even fun. Tips on taking pills, having x-rays, and dealing with IVs can help make these procedures go more smoothly. Decorating the hospital room and visiting play therapists will make your child's stay more cheerful. Your entire family's comfort and peace of mind will greatly increase once you've formed a close working relationship with your child's doctors and nurses. Knowing what to expect will help ease your fears and empower you to be a strong advocate for your child.

Being your child's advocate may be a new role for you. This book will help you work more effectively with medical personnel by discussing how to:

- **Make a plan.** Consider what to bring to the hospital, how to prepare your child, and ways to adjust your work schedule and deal with your child's schooling.

- **Educate yourself.** Learn all you can about the treatment, surgery, doctor, and hospital, and how to find materials to help prepare your child.

- **Communicate.** Work with family, friends, doctors, and nurses to build a team that will focus on your child's care. Help to ensure that your child's doctor hears your concerns and that you understand the doctor.

- **Be a role model.** Learn how other parents comforted their children and coped with behavior changes in their children during and after the trip to the hospital.

Every family is unique. Your child's hospital visit may be a whirlwind affair, while other children may be in the hospital for months. Because each family has different needs, this book presents a range of suggestions and stories. You will be able to pick, from hundreds of suggestions, the things that will best help your child. Don't expect to follow the advice of all forty parents—you will be overwhelmed rather than empowered. Think of the book as simply a rich menu of choices.

This book covers emergency room visits, short-term stays, and lengthy hospitalizations. Information that applies to all families is located at the beginning of each chapter. Specific suggestions for families whose children have serious injuries or long-term illnesses are offered separately, so that you can read only the parts that pertain to your particular situation.

In this second edition, we've added journal pages where children can express their feelings about their hospitalization through words or drawings. These journal pages can give children some control over the experience and allow parents insight into how the child is perceiving what's happening. After the hospital visit, the journal pages can help the visit be remembered more accurately, rather than becoming a hazy, strange, or frightening memory.

At the end of the book is a resource section that lists books for parents and children of all ages. Organizations that help families with hospitalizations are also included. A packing list compiled by veterans of many hospital stays will help you decide what to bring along.

You know your child best. With that knowledge and the advice from forty parents who have been there, you will be equipped to prepare your child for the trip to the hospital, get him better as quickly as possible, and then come home.

# CHAPTER ONE

# Before You Go

*If you face trouble sanely,*
*it cannot trouble you.*

—*Lao Tzu*

MOST PARENTS WOULD BE GLAD never to have to take their child to the hospital. Hospitals can be noisy, overwhelming places that frighten children (and sometimes parents). And hospital stays can be extraordinarily expensive, even when insurance coverage is good. But preparing well and getting the information you need before your child goes to the hospital can make the experience much easier for you, your child, and your family.

## Is hospitalization necessary?

In emergencies, you may not have time to ask your doctor questions about your child's hospitalization. But, in most circumstances, you can discuss with your doctor in advance the reasons for the hospitalization. Good planning includes asking some important questions when your doctor recommends hospitalization:

- Why is hospitalization necessary?

- Are there any alternatives such as outpatient surgery?

*When Claire had her tonsils out, they did it as an outpatient surgery. At first I was shocked that they were going to send my daughter home after just a few hours. Now I would insist on it whenever possible. I think it's almost always better to be at home if you can be. It's more cost effective and the child can benefit from a familiar environment and the comforts of home.*

- Who will perform the procedure or surgery?

- What are the risks, if any?

- Please explain the process in detail and in language that is understandable to me.

- Are books, pamphlets, or videos available that describe the procedure or surgery?

- Is there a child life specialist on staff who will help prepare my child?

- If not, are there experienced parents who can talk with me about how to prepare my child?

- Can I stay with my child during the procedure?

Try to get enough information to help you and your child prepare for medical treatments and procedures. Knowing what to expect will lower your anxiety level as well as your child's.

*When Ian's doctor recommended surgery to correct his eyes, which were starting to turn in, I was very reluctant to agree because Ian was so young. The doctor told me that without surgery, his eyes could get worse and would not be able to be treated in the future. I talked to a lot of other people and got a second opinion. At that point, we felt much more comfortable going ahead with the surgery.*

# Get a second opinion

Conscientious doctors welcome consultations and encourage second opinions. There are many gray areas in medicine where judgment and experience are as important as knowledge. Many insurance companies require a second opinion. If, after discussions with the doctor, you are still uneasy about any aspect of your child's medical care, do not hesitate to seek another opinion.

There are two ways to get a second opinion: see another specialist, or ask your child's specialist to arrange a multidisciplinary second opinion. Many parents get a second opinion before moving ahead with any but the most routine or emergency treatment. You do not need to do this in secret. Explain to your child's physician that, before proceeding, you would like a second opinion.

Try to find an independent physician to provide one; doctors who share a practice or regularly give referrals to each other may be leery of disagreeing with their colleagues. To allow for a thorough analysis, arrange to have copies of all records sent ahead to the physician who will give the second opinion.

Sometimes, with complex illnesses or injuries, a group of specialists will meet to review the case. Ask your doctor about this type of multidisciplinary review if you believe your child needs one.

Parents often hesitate suggesting a second opinion because they are afraid of offending the doctor or creating antagonism. Your child's doctor should not resent it if you seek a second opinion. If the doctor does resist, explain you need a second opinion in order to feel comfortable about proceeding with the treatment.

> *My daughter was having debilitating pain but her ob/gyn didn't seem concerned. When I asked how she was going to treat it, the doctor said, "Oh, she's just going to have to live with that." So, we called the Endometriosis Society and got the names of several specialists. I asked nurses that I knew who they would recommend and also called the ob/gyn floor at the hospital for recommendations. The same doctor's name was on everyone's list. We have been going to her now for ten years. She is absolutely wonderful and means the world to us.*

# Find a specialist

Often a hospitalized child will need a specialist to perform surgery, give anesthesia, or provide other treatment. Your choice of specialists may be limited by the hospital, time constraints, and insurance or HMO restrictions. Usually, your child's primary physician recommends an appropriate specialist. Make sure that your insurance will cover the specialist you choose.

The following list may help you feel more comfortable with the recommended specialist. If you have time, try to make sure that your child's specialist:

• Is board-certified. This means that the specialist has passed rigorous written and oral tests administered by a board of examiners in his specialty. You can call the American Board of Medical Specialties at 1-800-776-2378 to find out if the specialist is board-certified.

• Establishes a good rapport with your child.

• Communicates clearly and compassionately.

• Answers all questions using language that is easy to understand.

• Consults with other doctors about complex problems.

• Makes all test results available.

• Is willing to let you participate in the decision-making process.

• Respects your values.

Often the specialist the primary doctor recommends is a good match and the family finds him easy to communicate with, competent, and caring. If you don't develop a good rapport with the specialist initially recommended to you, ask for or locate another physician.

# Make a plan

Begin planning your child's hospitalization as soon as you establish that it is necessary. Even a brief hospital stay can be physically draining and emotionally difficult, so take time before the visit to prepare your child and family.

• Research the proposed medical procedure or surgery. Often a friend or family member can help you find the best doctor, hospital, and medical team to perform the surgery or procedure. Make yourself a knowledgeable part of the medical team.

- Arrange care for your other children. This should be with someone they know and like who can help the siblings carry on with their normal routine (school, lessons, sports). Also, child care should be flexible in case you need to stay longer than planned at the hospital.

- Plan how you will keep your household functioning. Find a friend or neighbor to feed animals, water the plants, and pick up mail.

- Take time off work and school. Talk with your child's teacher about ways to keep your child current while he is hospitalized.

- Make a list of names and telephone numbers of people you can call on for help. Sometimes you can designate one person to call others to share news, coordinate food, or baby-sit.

- Find out what equipment and services the hospital has available, such as play rooms, refrigerators for parents' food, or special long-term parking.

- Pack ahead of time. Sometimes your child can help choose clothes, toys, and books to bring to the hospital. (Use the *Packing List* in the back of this book to get ideas on what to bring.)

- Plan how you will prepare your child and his siblings for the visit.

*My daughter has been hospitalized twice to control her seizures. To prepare, I went to the library and took out every book they had on seizure disorders. I asked the neurologist if he had any books to recommend. Then I went to the school nurse and asked her to give other parents of children who had seizures my name and telephone number. I contacted the Epilepsy Foundation and they sent loads of literature plus a list of people to contact. Talking to the other parents and reading books really helped us plan her medical care.*

Consider whether your child might be helped by a hospital tour, a talk with the doctor, or a chat with other patients who have undergone similar treatment. You might visit the library to find books about your child's illness or injury or about hospital stays. (The *Resources* section in the back of this book contains suggested reading.)

*We had a wonderful relationship with the oncologist assigned to us. He blended perfectly the science and art of medicine. His manner was warm, he was extremely qualified professionally, and he was very easy to talk with. He welcomed discussions about articles I brought in. Although he was busy, we never felt rushed. I laughed when I saw that he had written in the chart, "Mother asks innumerable appropriate questions."*

# CHAPTER TWO

# The Emergency Room

*The best way out is always through.*

—*Robert Frost*

DOCTORS IN EMERGENCY ROOMS treat serious trauma and illnesses every day. Often, especially on Friday and Saturday nights, the emergency room is full. Doctors and nurses in emergency rooms work under stressful conditions and may not have time to make your visit comfortable. Consequently, medical care may seem impersonal. And during very busy times, treatment for conditions that aren't life-threatening may be slow.

## Avoid the emergency room

Try to avoid the emergency room whenever possible. Your family doctor or a walk-in clinic often may treat you more quickly and efficiently than an emergency room. And your family doctor is more familiar and probably less expensive.

Many parents also try to avoid taking their child to the hospital in an ambu-

*One evening my three-year-old, Gylany, fell off the couch, hit her head on the floor, and passed out for a few seconds. I scooped her up, grabbed my five-year-old, and went to the ER. We checked in, then waited for over two hours. My kids were exhausted from crying. Whenever I asked the receptionist how long it would be, she said, "They will be right with you." Gylany threw up, and we still waited a half hour before they finally saw us. We were there until one thirty in the morning. It was horrible.*

lance. In some areas, public ambulance service is free; in other regions, the shortest of ambulance rides can cost hundreds of dollars. Do not drive yourself if the emergency is life-threatening, if your child may require treatment during transport, or if you are too worried to drive safely. When in doubt, call an ambulance.

## Call your doctor

Call your doctor before you go to the emergency room if time allows. She may be able to suggest a treatment option that helps you avoid the emergency room altogether. If you must go, your doctor may be able to meet you there. In addition to a comforting presence, your doctor can provide a second opinion, a referral, or pertinent information about your child's medical history.

*One day I got a call at work; Patrick had fallen and cut open his chin. I immediately called our local family practice doctor. He told us to go to the ER and he would meet us there. We trusted the doctor not to keep us waiting. The personal connection also meant we were treated less like a number.*

It can also help to bring your spouse or another adult who acts as an advocate while you comfort your child. The advocate can call family or employers, fill out paperwork, and ask questions. Having another adult present allows you to stay at your child's side so that you can attend to her needs.

## Bring something to do

Emergency rooms pick the most urgent cases to treat first. Depending on the emergency room's patient load and your child's needs, you may wait hours for treatment.

Even if you have just a moment before bringing your child in, try to grab something to comfort and distract your child: a stuffed animal, a familiar book, some crayons, or a computer game. If you don't have time to bring something, ask at the emergency room desk. Many ER's keep some toys on hand for just such occasions.

You should also try to explain to your child what will happen during the visit. Even if you don't know the details, you can explain that the doctor will conduct an examination and do whatever is possible to make her feel better.

## Stay with your child

Whenever your child goes to the emergency room, she should have a reassuring parent present if possible. At times, staff will try to keep you out of treatment areas. Doctors and nurses worry that you will get in their way or further agitate your child. If you are very emotional, these may be valid concerns. However, you usually can insist on staying with your child if you are calm. Use your judgment—if your child is unconscious or has suffered severe trauma, you may choose to wait outside.

But most injuries and illnesses are not severe, and your child will probably draw more comfort from having you present than anyone else. You can provide great reassurance by holding your child's hand, singing, or quietly explaining what's happening.

When you arrive in an emergency room, you must fill out paperwork, including medical history and insurance information. This can be time-consuming and, if your child is seriously injured, hospital staff will want to begin treatment immediately. You can ask your spouse or a friend to handle the paperwork, or take it into the exam room.

> *While the doctor manipulated the broken bone, I kept bodily contact with Aurora. I stroked what I could. At one point, I held her foot. It helped her be calm and feel connected. I stood at her foot when they were working by her head. I stayed where they weren't.*

## Working with staff

It's a good idea to establish rapport with emergency room staff right away. That means staying calm, asking questions, providing accurate information, and gently but regularly making staff aware of your presence. Prior to giving permission for medications, make sure you tell the staff about any prescription or over-the-counter drugs that your child takes, for example, an asthma inhaler or an antihistamine.

Politely ask the doctors what they are doing and why. Try to understand the treatment plan for your child's illness or injury. If you are uneasy about the proposed treatment, ask for another opinion. In large teaching hospitals, the first doctor you see usually is a resident. Ask to see a chief resident or attending physician if you feel another opinion is necessary (the different types of doctors in teaching hospitals are explained in Chapter 5, *Telling the Staff Apart.*

If your child will be going home with you, ask for all instructions in writing—you may not remember later. You might also ask about:

- Possible complications related to medication.

- Effects, such as swelling or fevers, that might occur later and when you should call about such symptoms.

- Special care for stitches, bandages, or casts.

- Whether you should call your primary physician to arrange for follow-up care.

Do not hesitate to call the emergency room or your family physician if something appears amiss with your child when you come home.

> One night, we took our eighteen-month-old daughter, who has diabetes, to the ER because of a sudden, severe ear infection. I had already checked her blood sugar and it was fine. But when they heard "diabetes," they immediately began to draw blood and put a urine bag on her. I said, "Stop for a moment and listen to me." After I explained, they just dealt with the infection.

# Be a role model

Your child looks to you for clues about how to act. If you are emotionally distraught or squeamish, your child will be more likely to get upset in the emergency room. Do your best to remain calm and strong. If the sight of blood disturbs you, look away. If you feel faint, put your head between your knees or leave the room.

Many parents can hold their emotions in check until their child is out of danger. But don't be surprised if you feel the need to cry when it's all over.

*She broke her right wrist and it caused what they call significant deformation. It was really gross. But while the doctor worked on it, I tried to not register alarm or shock. I kept real impassive features so if she were trying to read my face, I would be more or less inscrutable. When it's my kid and I don't want to scare her, I click into warrior mom.*

# Staying in the hospital

Sometimes a child is too seriously ill or injured to go home after an emergency room visit. Doctors then will recommend that your child be admitted to the hospital. Your child will be moved to another floor and placed in a room, sometimes alone, sometimes with other children. You can always ask if a single room is available. You might check with your insurance company to find out whether a private room will be covered if it's not medically necessary.

Again, try to remain with your child if he is admitted. Use the telephone in the room to notify your work and family. If you left the house without clothes, toys, or books for your child, find someone to collect these items and bring them to the hospital. Also, have them bring a change of clothes and toothbrush for you if you are spending the night.

When your child settles in, a nurse probably will come into the room, start a chart, and take vital signs (blood pressure, heart rate, breathing rate). The nurse may ask you to repeat information that you already gave to the emergency room staff. This may seem repetitive, but ER staff often abbreviate the information you provide. You may also have forgotten an important detail in the emergency room. It's important for both you and your child's caregivers to provide information and answer questions.

The nurse also should explain what will happen that night. For example, if your child has a concussion, the nurse may need to wake her up every hour. If the nurse doesn't explain the first night's plan, do not hesitate to ask.

# CHAPTER THREE

# Preparing Your Child

*What can I know? What should I do?*
*What may I hope?*

—*Immanuel Kant*

CHILDREN WHO ARE WELL PREPARED for hospital visits feel comfortable and sometimes even excited about their upcoming hospitalization. Children who aren't expecting the strange surroundings or discomfort of medical procedures can be more difficult to work with and may have residual emotional trauma after they leave.

## Help from hospital staff

You can find many resources in your doctor's office, at the library, or at the hospital to help prepare your child for his hospital visit. Some doctors provide videos that explain surgery and other procedures in terms children understand.

Many children's hospitals employ child life specialists who can help your child act out a procedure using dolls and play instruments. Hospitals also have social workers and counselors skilled at explaining how hospitals

> *Matthew was in sixth grade and he was worried about the surgery for putting in the catheter. The child life worker showed him what a catheter looked like, then they explored the pre-op area, the actual surgery room, and post-op. She showed him on a cloth doll exactly where the incision would be and how the scar would look. Then she introduced him to "Fred," the IV pump. She said that Fred would be going places with him, and that Fred would keep him from getting so many pokes. She really helped him with his fears.*

work and answering your child's questions. As soon as you know your child will be spending time in the hospital, ask your doctor about these specialized services.

## Taking a tour

A tour can be an excellent way to familiarize your child with hospital surroundings before admission. The tour might include a look at the operating room, an explanation of anesthesia, and an opportunity to talk with children who have undergone similar procedures.

During a tour or at some other pre-arranged time, try to take your child to meet the people who will provide her care, including doctors, nurses, surgeons, and anesthesiologists. Children are less afraid of adults they know; and doctors and nurses often form attachments to children they have met.

If you take a tour, make sure your child also gets to see the fun parts of the hospital, such as the play area and cafeteria. Although adults often cringe at hospital cafeteria food, many children enjoy walking through the line and choosing their own food.

*Eighteen-month-old Gylany had the croup. Our pediatrician sent her to the hospital to spend the night in a humidified tent. I told her, "We're going to have an adventure today. We are going to the hospital to get some help for your breathing. We're going to camp out in a tent there. It will be just like the rain forest, but instead of raining on the outside of the tent it will rain on the inside. I'll stay with you and we'll cuddle in our tent, and look for rain forest birds and animals." I climbed right into the tent and we spent the night in our private rain forest.*

It also helps to tell your child some of the positive things about going to the hospital.

- He will not have to make his bed, do his chores, or wash the dishes.

- She will get her own telephone, television, and remote control.

- He will get to pick his own food off a menu and eat in bed.

- She will have buttons to push that make the bed go up and down.

Show your child that all beds in the hospital—even adults' beds—have rails on the sides.

You might also make the tour part of an educational experience. If your child will return to school shortly after the hospitalization, you or your child can talk to his teacher about letting him do a report or research project on some aspect of hospital life. Asking questions and becoming something of a hospital expert may help your child feel more informed and in control of the situation.

# Reading books together

Try to find several age-appropriate books to read with your child. Books offer factual information that may clear up any misconceptions or fears your child has about what happens at the hospital. Reading together also allows time for your child to ask you questions and perhaps share some worries.

You can find helpful books at your local bookstore. They usually have a children's book expert who knows what's available for each age group. The hospital social worker, counselor, or child life specialist may also have recommendations. Many suggestions are listed in the *Resources* section at the end of this book.

*When my son was preparing to go to the hospital, we bought a book written by Mr. Rogers, called* Going to the Hospital. *It showed children and their families in the hospital, during admission, having x-rays, in bed. It was very reassuring and informative. Reading books allowed his fears and concerns to surface. He asked questions he might not have asked if we hadn't cuddled up on the couch and read the book together.*

# Answering questions

Whether you use books, videos, tours, or other methods to prepare your child, it helps to check her understanding. Children sometimes believe they are going to the hospital as punishment. Explain that this is not the case; tell your child that hospitals are special places that help people who are hurt or sick.

Children also form incorrect impressions or have fearful fantasies about what can occur. They can conjure up genuine horrors and you should try to replace those fearful imaginings with the truth.

> Our children perceive things differently than we do. We've found it's really important to ask them to explain to us what they think is coming. A lot of times we can dispel their fears. Before heart surgeries, we have asked David what he thinks is going to happen. Once he asked, "How do I know they're not going to take my heart out?"

Be realistic. If you tell your child that a painful procedure won't hurt, he won't believe you the next time. Be truthful, and explain the procedure as well as you can. Consider letting your child ask the doctor questions, too.

To answer questions, you must inform yourself: read books, talk to staff, and chat with parents and children who have undergone similar treatment.

If your child is very young, she will be unable to ask questions or understand explanations. An infant's whole world is eating, sleeping, being held, being sung to, and being nestled in his parent's arms. These familiar comforts will help soothe your baby during medical procedures.

# Help with longer-term treatment

If your child will be in the hospital or undergoing medical treatments for a prolonged period, a child life worker can do a great deal to help your child understand and deal with the hospital and medical treatment. Child life professionals provide play experiences

> *For Christie, playing "procedures" helped release many feelings. We stocked a medical kit with gauze pads, tape, tubing, stethoscope, reflex hammer, and pretend needles and syringes. We made IV bottles from empty shampoo containers, complete with tubing and plastic needles. Many dolls and stuffed animals in our house fell apart after being speared by the pen during countless spinal taps.*

that encourage expression of feelings and increase understanding. They also communicate with other members of the health care team about the psychosocial needs of children and their families.

Coping with procedures is especially important for frequently hospitalized children. Many child life specialists accompany children to procedures and stay to provide support.

You can discuss when and how to prepare your child for upcoming procedures with the child life professional or hospital social worker. Consider how much advance notice to give your child before procedures. You may want to experiment. Some children do better with several days to prepare, while others just spend the time worrying. Sometimes, a child's needs change as treatment progresses, so good communication and flexibility are essential.

> *Ian was cross-eyed. We had a couple of friends who had eye procedures done. They both talked to him and told him how much better they were after surgery. They really set up a feeling of "I've been through this. It was fine. It was an okay experience to go through it." It helped him a lot.*

Giving children some control over what happens helps tremendously. Children have definite opinions about how they want things done in the hospital. Encourage your child to express those opinions and do what you can to accommodate them. For example, your child might prefer that you hold her during a procedure, instead of a nurse.

One or both parents should try to be present during all procedures, especially for small children. Parents set the tone. A calm parent and a well-prepared child create the best atmosphere for a quick, peaceful procedure. If you find that you are unable to help your child, ask the child life specialist or other member of the health care team to be present solely to comfort your child.

Many clinics have a special box full of toys for children who have had a procedure. It may help for your child to have a treat to look forward to.

# CHAPTER FOUR

# The Facilities

*Remember that worry will cause much pain
over things that will never happen.*

—*Thomas Jefferson*

WHETHER YOU AND YOUR CHILD are in the hospital for a day or for much longer, the experience can be trying. Hospitals are huge bureaucracies—noisy, impersonal, and running on a time schedule all their own. For a child, being hospitalized means being separated from parents, brothers, sisters, friends, pets, and the comfort and familiarity of home. A child's hospitalization can sometimes make parents and child feel vulnerable and helpless. But with a little ingenuity, you can make the most of the facilities, liven up the atmosphere, and even have some fun.

## Staying with your child

One of the biggest worries a child has in the hospital is being separated from his parents. If you stay at your child's side, you can provide comfort, protection, and advocacy.

The majority of pediatric hospitals know how much better most children do when a parent sleeps in the room.

> *My daughter is now a young adult, but she has had several major surgeries since she was 15. Generally, the nurses tell me that I cannot stay with her in the room overnight because she is old enough to take care of herself. Well, I'm a nurse, and in our family, whether you are an adult or child, someone stays with you in the hospital around the clock. So, I just nicely tell them, "I will be quiet, I won't get in your way. As a matter of fact, I'll help out quite a bit. But I am going to stay." And I do.*

Sometimes small couches convert into beds, or you can use a cot provided by the hospital. If hospital policy requires you to leave, negotiate with the hospital administrator. You may also be able to get support from your primary doctor.

Sometimes it isn't possible to stay with your child if you are a single parent or if both parents work full time. Many families have grandparents, aunts and uncles, or close friends who stay at the hospital when parents cannot be present. Older children and teenagers may not want a parent in the room at night, but they need an advocate there during the day just as much as younger children.

*A couple of years ago, David said, "I'm not going through another heart surgery." We said, "You talk with the doctor." He talked to the doctor, who told him he'd be able to run faster and ride his bike. Since he was the slowest runner in his class, being able to run faster was a big deal. So he agreed to go through with the surgery.*

You can teach children who are old enough to use the telephone for times when a family member cannot be present. Tape a phone number nearby where you can be reached and instruct your child to call if anyone proposes an unexpected change in treatment. Tell hospital staff that only you can authorize such changes, unless the situation is life-threatening.

Illness and hospitals can make children feel like their bodies are being invaded. Your child may feel better if you take responsibility for some nursing care. Children usually prefer parents to help them to the bathroom or to change dirty sheets. If you can make the bed, keep the room tidy, change dressings, and give back rubs, you will free nurses to spend more time providing medical care for your child.

If you encourage your child to make choices whenever possible, you may help him regain a sense of personal power.

- Older children should be included in all discussions about their treatment.

- Younger children can decide when to take a bath, which arm to use for an IV, what to order for meals, what clothes to wear, and how to decorate the room.

- Some children request a hug or a handshake after all treatments or procedures.

# The room

Hospital rooms often are painted drab colors, and most rooms don't have particularly scenic views. You (and your child if he is well enough) can do a lot to liven up a dull hospital room. If your child's hospital visit will be brief, a few touches of home probably will suffice. If the visit will be longer, more extensive efforts to make the room more familiar and welcoming may be in order.

- Cover the walls with big, bright posters (Disney characters, sports figures, rock groups).

- Tape cards on the walls, hang them from strings like a mobile, or arrange them around the windowsills.

- Attach crepe paper streamers to the ceiling.

- Put up pictures of the child engaged in her favorite activity. Add photos of family members, friends, and pets.

- Bring bouquets of balloons (Mylar) and leave them bobbing in the corners.

- Place a favorite stuffed animal, blanket, or quilt on the bed. This can

> *The first thing we did was put up a poster of the Little Engine that Could saying, "I think I can. I think I can." Then we covered every square inch of the walls of three-year-old Meagan's room with colorful posters. We tried to use ones with depth so it would seem like the room was larger. We hung up all of her cards from her preschool friends. Balloons covered the ceiling. The room was colorful and full.*

provide great comfort, especially for younger children. You may have to make sure your linens or animals are not accidentally carted away with the soiled linens.

- Make the room smell good with potpourri or aromatherapy oils if smells don't bother your child.

- Bring a guest book for each visitor and member of the medical staff to sign. Or put up a sign-in poster for doctors and nurses, who must sign in before they begin examinations or take vital signs. Some parents ask staff members to outline their hands on a poster and write inside the print.

- Place a journal in the child's room for visitors, family members, doctors, and nurses to write in.

*My daughter's preschool teacher sent a care package. She made a felt board with dozens of cutout characters and designs that provided hours of quiet entertainment. She also included games, drawings from each classmate, coloring books, markers, get well cards, and a child's tape player with earphones. Because we had run out of our house with just the clothes on our backs, all of these toys were very, very welcome.*

- Bring music to block out hospital noise and help everyone relax. A small cassette player, Walkman with earphones, or CD boom box is portable and useful.

- Bring clothes from home. Many hospitals provide brightly colored smocks for young patients, but many children and teens prefer to wear their own clothing. This can pose a laundry problem, so check to see if the floor has washers available for families.

- Sign up for a VCR if the hospital has them. Bring in or rent a favorite or funny video. Humor helps.

- Bring in age-appropriate games, puzzles, and books.

Ask for a tour of the floor as soon as possible after admission. Find out if a microwave and refrigerator are available; ask about sleeping arrangements for parents, and discuss showers and bathtubs for patients and parents. Obtain a hospital handbook if one is available. These booklets often include information on billing, parking, discounts, and other helpful tips.

# Where do the kids play?

*When I wanted to have a conference with the doctor about Katy's treatment, I called recreation therapy and they sent two wonderful ladies to the clinic. The doctor and I were able to talk privately for an hour, and Katy had a great time making herself a gold crown and decorating her wheelchair with streamers and jewels.*

Children need to play, especially when hospitalized. Ask whether the hospital has a recreation therapy department. Often, a large room is devoted to toys, books, dolls, and crafts, and is staffed by specialists who have training in play therapy. These rooms provide many therapeutic activities, such as medical play with dolls, as well as art materials, building blocks, crafts, and music.

Recreation therapy encourages contact with other children in similar circumstances and helps children feel less alone. Most important, the recreation therapy rooms are a cheerful change from lying in a hospital bed. They are full of fun activities and smiling staff people.

If a child is immobile or too ill to go to the play area, arrangements can be made for a recreation therapist to bring a bundle of toys, games, and books to the room. This can give you time to go out to eat or take a walk.

Exercise also is important.

- Kids who are strong enough to walk can have a great time exploring the hospital. Plan a daily excursion to the gift shop or the cafeteria. Go outside and walk the hospital perimeter if weather and the neighborhood allow.

- Treat mechanical devices, such as crutches or IV poles, as playthings rather than hindrances. It's not unusual to see small children standing on the base of an IV pole and hanging on while a parent pushes the pole down the hall at a rapid clip.

- Check to see if the hospital has a swimming pool; if your child can't use it, you probably can.

*I do not allow more than two people in the room at a time and Apryl makes sure they wash their hands. Most of the residents who have been there awhile know of my quirks, but these quirks are there to protect Apryl which is of more importance than making the interns and students happy.*

## Food

The hospital will provide meals for your child. But you must eat as well and buying meals day after day in the hospital cafeteria can get expensive.

- Check to see if the floor has a refrigerator, microwave, or kitchen for patient use. Since children often want to eat between meals, such facilities are handy to heat hot chocolate, make popcorn, or cook leftovers.

- Put your name in a prominent place on your containers.

- Ask family members and friends to bring food when they visit.

- Find out which local restaurants deliver take-out food to hospital rooms.

- Consider ordering extra items to come up on your child's tray.

## Parking

Emergency areas typically have special parking spots in front of the entrance. But finding regular parking near hospitals can be difficult. Many parents have unpleasant memories of driving around in endless loops looking for a parking space with their sick child sitting in the back seat. Ask about parking arrangements for long stays or regular visits. Find out whether parking passes are available or where the cheapest parking is located.

# The hospital waiting game

You can expect lengthy waits for everything from routine tests to surgery. Many parents find themselves getting nervous or angry in large teaching hospitals while waiting for the doctors to appear during rounds each morning (when attending physicians, residents, and interns move from room to room in a large group); then feel let down when the visit lasts only a few moments. If you have questions, write them down and tell the doctors when they come in that you would like a few moments to talk with them.

Some young patients become upset when large groups of doctors or nurses come in during rounds. If this bothers your child, request that only your doctor and assigned nurse be admitted. You have the right to refuse student doctors if you feel that their presence is not helpful for your child.

Even if your child is in a community hospital, you may have to wait for the doctor. If you become frustrated, call his office to get an estimate on when he will arrive.

The hospital may have VCRs and games available in waiting rooms, but usually you need to bring your own things. Have your child pick out favorite card games, board games, computer games, drawing materials, and books. You can bring food and drinks as long as they don't interfere with your child's treatment plan.

*It seemed like we spent most of the years of treatment waiting to see a doctor who was running hours behind schedule, so I came well prepared. I always carried a large bag containing an assortment of things to eat and drink, toys to play with, coloring books and markers, books to read, and Play-Doh. My son stayed occupied and we avoided many problems. I saw too many parents in the waiting room expecting their bored children to sit still and be quiet for long periods of time.*

# CHAPTER FIVE

# Telling the Staff Apart

*It is one of the most beautiful compensations of this
life that no man can sincerely try to help
another without helping himself.*

—*Ralph Waldo Emerson*

IN LARGE HOSPITALS, a steady parade of anonymous faces passes through the life of a hospitalized child. Understanding the hospital hierarchy can help you sort out who is responsible for your child's care.

## The doctors

As with any other profession, doctors have many different specialties, temperaments, and skill levels. Your child's treatment will be greatly enhanced if you and your child trust and communicate well with your doctor. The majority of discussions and decision-making will take place with the primary care doctor and your child's specialist.

- **Primary physician.** Your child's primary physician (usually a pediatrician or family practice doctor) oversees all medical care. When your child is in the hospital, the primary physician often will visit, get reports from specialists, and check on your child. The primary physician also should be available to answer questions and provide support.

- **Specialist.** A specialist has extensive training in a specific area of medicine. Cardiologists, for example, specialize in hearts; orthopedists specialize in bones and joints.

Along with the doctors you choose, your child may see many other doctors if he is in a teaching hospital.

- **Medical student.** A medical student is a college graduate who is attending medical school. Medical students wear white coats, but do not have M.D. on their name tags.

- **Intern.** An intern (sometimes called a first-year resident) is a graduate of medical school who is in the first year of postgraduate training.

- **Resident.** A resident is a graduate of medical school in her second to sixth year of postgraduate training. Most residents at pediatric hospitals will be pediatricians upon completion of their residencies.

- **Fellow.** A fellow is a doctor who has completed four years of medical school, several years of residency, and is taking additional specialty training.

- **Attending physician.** An attending physician (called simply "attending") is above a fellow in the hospital hierarchy. Medical centers hire these well-established doctors to provide and oversee medical care and to train interns, residents, and fellows. They are frequently also professors on the staff of an affiliated medical school.

If your child is at a community hospital, her primary doctor will provide most of her care. But if your child is at a teaching hospital, she will be assigned a doctor from the appropriate specialty. These physicians will care for your child throughout treatment. The physician in charge of your child's care should be board-certified or have equivalent medical credentials.

If your child is a patient at a teaching hospital, he will see a large number of other doctors. Residents usually rotate to different floors every four weeks, so they are an ever-changing group. The fellow or attending assigned to your child will be most familiar with your child's situation and is the best person to seek out if questions arise about your child's treatment or illness.

# The nurses

The nursing staff is an essential part of the hospital hierarchy. Several nurses with different levels of training all may play a role in your child's treatment.

- **Nurse assistant or aide.** A nurse assistant can take vital signs (heart rate, breathing rate, blood pressure), perform hygiene care, or help with mobility.

- **Licensed practical nurse (LPN).** An LPN has completed a vocational training program and has a narrow scope of practice. LPNs take vital signs, give medications, and perform general care under the supervision of a registered nurse.

> At our hospital, each of our nurses is different, but each is wonderful. They simply love the kids. They listen to the kids, throw parties, set up dream trips, act as counselor, best friend, stern parent. They hug moms and dads. They cry. I have come to respect them so much because they have such a hard job to do, and they do it so well.

- **Registered nurse (RN).** An RN receives a bachelor's or associate's degree in nursing, then takes a licensing examination. These medical professionals give medicines, take vital signs, start and monitor IVs, communicate changes in condition to doctors, change bandages, and care for patients in hospitals, clinics, and doctor's offices.

- **Nurse practitioner or clinical nurse specialist.** A nurse practitioner is a registered nurse who has completed an educational program that covers advanced skills. In some hospitals and clinics, nurse practitioners perform procedures, such as spinal taps.

- **Head nurse or charge nurse.** A head nurse supervises all the nurses on the floor for one shift.

- **Clinical nurse manager.** A clinical nurse manager is the administrator for an entire floor, unit, or clinic.

Working closely with nurses is the unit secretary. The unit secretary has many duties, including answering call buttons and relaying requests to nurses, answering the telephone, and transcribing all doctors' orders.

# Befriending the staff

Many wonderful and some not-so-wonderful people staff hospitals. Parents sometimes find that their anxiety makes them less tolerant of inefficiency or confusion. Your child will feel more secure if you work with hospital staff rather than becoming adversarial. If you help change your child's soiled bedding, take out food trays, and give baths, you will free overworked nurses to take care of medicines and IVs. Nurses really appreciate the help and usually reciprocate by answering questions or negotiating with doctors for you.

*Give staff a chance to see your child as a human being. Show pictures. "This is the little kid who likes Barney. He loves to play this song. This is what he looks like when he's not all puffed up from surgery." They see so many kids who are so sick every day. It's important for them to see that sparkle in your child's eye.*

Some parents recommend introducing themselves and their child to the nurse and residents on each shift. You might add that you'll help as much as you can. If they are not too busy, talk with them about matters unrelated to the hospital. Establishing a personal relationship makes everyone feel more comfortable and connected. Try to thank them for any kind words or deeds.

# Shift changes

As soon as you can, learn about the shift changes on your child's floor. These generally occur every eight or twelve hours. Resentments can begin when parents don't understand what happens during shift changes.

Shift change is a necessary, and sometimes hectic, organization time for the nurses to plan how to best deliver care for the next eight to twelve hours. During a shift change, the outgoing staff meet with the incoming staff to report on the status of all the patients on the floor. They discuss:

- A brief history of each patient.

- A summary of major events from the last two shifts, such as, "She vomited after each dose of morphine, so today we switched to Tylenol with codeine and she's feeling much better."

- What needs to be done, for example, "The lab work is not done yet and Dr. Jones is waiting for the results."

- Family information, such as, "His father had to go to work. The telephone number there is posted by the bed. His aunt is staying with him now."

> *Whenever Kathryn is hospitalized, I introduce myself and my daughter and ask when the shift change is. Then I say, "I'll do my best not to bother you." I always get a grateful smile. If I need something and I see them in report, I wave and go back into the room. I get more smiles. Then, whenever I really need help, they are almost always just fabulous. I've found that when we all work as a team, it goes much smoother.*

After hearing a report on all the patients, the nurses decide how to assign patients to incoming nurses to keep the work load even. Next, each nurse spends a few minutes organizing and prioritizing what he needs to do for each of his patients.

You should try not to call during the shift change hour (a half hour before and a half hour after) with any non-urgent questions, comments, or requests. If you press the call button, the unit secretary will tell you it may be a while before a nurse comes because, "They are in report." Of course, the nurses will respond to things that cannot wait, such as your child vomiting, an empty IV bag, severe pain, or another emergency.

# CHAPTER SIX

# Communicating with Staff

*In necessary things, unity; in doubtful things,*
*liberty; in all things, charity.*

—*St. Augustine*

COMMUNICATING WELL WITH YOUR DOCTOR can mean the difference between a very good relationship and a very poor one. Good communication can improve your child's care and put your mind at ease. Poor communication can leave doctors, parents, and children feeling angry and resentful.

## Types of relationships

There are three types of relationships that typically develop between physicians and parents: authoritarian, collegial, or adversarial. Most doctors have one preferred style, authoritarian or collegial. Many switch between a more authoritarian or collegial role, depending on input from the patient.

- **Authoritarian.** In an authoritarian relationship, the doctor assumes a parental role and the child's family is submissive. Even though this kind of care can seem reassuring, doctors are human and, although they don't intend harm, mistakes occur. If parents place blind faith in medical staff and do not monitor drugs and treatments, these mistakes may go unnoticed. Parents need to become the experts on their own child and pay close attention to his reactions to drugs and treatments.

  Many parents stay in authoritarian relationships because they are intimidated by doctors and express the fear that if they question the doctors, their child will suffer. This type of behavior robs the child of an adult advocate who speaks up when something seems wrong.

- **Collegial.** A collegial relationship is a true partnership in which parents and caregivers are on the same footing and respect each other's domains and expertise. Here the doctor recognizes that many parents are experts on their own child. Parents respect the physician's knowledge and feel comfortable discussing treatment options or concerns that arise.

All parties must communicate honestly for this partnership to work, but the effort is worth it. Children develop confidence in their doctors, parents lessen their stress by creating a supportive relationship with the physician, and physicians feel comfortable that the family will comply with the treatment plan.

*Early in my daughter's treatment, we changed pediatricians. The first was aloof and patronizing, and the second was smart, warm, funny, and caring. He was a constant bright spot in our lives through some dark times. So every year, my two daughters put on their Santa hats and bring homemade cookies to the pediatrician and nurse. The first year I had to carry her in. She looked them in the eye and sang, "We Wish You a Merry Christmas." Her nurse went in the back room and cried, and her doctor got misty-eyed. I'll always be thankful for their care.*

- **Adversarial.** In an adversarial relationship, parents adopt an "us versus them" attitude that is counterproductive. Parents act as though the disease and any discomforts related to treatment are the fault of medical staff, and they blame staff for any setbacks that occur. This attitude undermines the child's confidence in his doctor, a crucial component for healing.

# Building rapport

Some parents want to know every detail of their child's treatment; others do not. As part of their preparation for hospitalization, parents should consider how much they want to know from hospital staff. Nurses and doctors cannot read parents' minds, nor can parents prepare their child for a procedure unless it has been explained well.

- Tell the staff how much you want to know.

- Inform staff of your child's temperament, likes, and dislikes.

- Encourage a close relationship between your child and his doctor. Insist that all medical personnel respect the young person's dignity. Do not let anyone talk in front of your child as if she is not there.

- Try to form a warm relationship with your child's nurse. Most children's hospitals assign each patient a primary nurse who will oversee all care. Nurses usually possess vast knowledge and experience about both medical and practical aspects of treatment. Often, nurses can rectify misunderstandings between doctor and parents.

- Ask for definitions of unfamiliar terms. Repeat back the information to ensure that you understood correctly. Don't hesitate to write down answers or tape-record conferences. If taping, it is helpful to say, "I hope you don't mind, but I have trouble remembering all of the information. This will help me keep everything straight." That way, the doctors are not put on the defensive and you have accomplished what you need.

- Take a written list of questions to appointments. This keeps you from forgetting something important and saves the staff from numerous follow-up phone calls.

- Ask questions only of your child's own physician whenever possible. Residents, fellows, or the on-call

*I told them the first day to treat me like a medical student. I asked them to share all information, current studies, lab results, everything, with me. I told them, in advance, that I hoped they wouldn't be offended by lots of questions, because knowledge was comfort to me.*

doctor may not be as familiar with the details of your child's condition.

- Make sure you know what medication or treatment is scheduled for each day. Make the final checks on all drugs whenever possible (check that it is the right drug, the correct dosage, and that your child's name is on the syringe or bag).

- Seek the best staff person to perform a procedure. The medical team includes many specialists: doctors, nurses, physical therapists, nutritionists, x-ray technicians, and more. At training hospitals, many of these people will be in the early stages of their careers. If a procedure is not going well, you can tell the person to stop and ask for a more skilled person to do the job.

> *We found that sitting down and talking things over with the nurses helped immensely. They were very familiar with each drug and its side effects. They told us many stories about children who had been through the same thing and were doing well years later. They always seemed to have time to give encouragement, a smile, or a hug.*

- Know your rights. Legally, your child cannot be treated without your permission. If a doctor proposes a procedure that you do not feel comfortable with, keep asking questions until you feel fully informed. You have the right to refuse the procedure if you do not think it is necessary. However, if the hospital staff feels that you are wrongfully withholding permission for treatment (if you reject standard treatment in favor of an unproven remedy, for example, or you are so concerned about side effects that you are endangering your child's well-being) they can take you to court. The child's health is at issue and both the hospital and the parents have input once you step into the legal arena.

## Improving communication

A positive relationship between parents and doctors thrives on clear and frequent communication. Doctors should explain clearly and listen well, and parents should feel comfortable asking questions and expressing concerns before they become grievances.

- Treat doctors with respect, and expect respect from them.

- Treat staff members with sensitivity. Recognize that you are under stress; so are doctors and nurses. Do not blame them for your child's illness or explode in anger. Be an advocate, not an adversary.

- Do not let problems build up until there is a long list of grievances. If you find yourself repeatedly asking hospital staff to fix the same problem seek a simple, practical solution that might benefit everyone involved.

- Request a conference if you have something to discuss with the doctor that will take time. These are routinely scheduled between parents and physicians, and should allow enough time for a thorough discussion. Grabbing a busy doctor in the hallway is unfair to him, and may result in an unsatisfactory answer to you.

- Negotiate. You have a right to a conversation with the doctor about your wishes. Tell her what you would like to see happen, and discuss all of the options. You may be able to work out a mutually acceptable plan.

- Do not be afraid to make waves if you believe you are right.

- Try to be genuinely friendly and helpful. Then, if a problem arises or you need help, your good relationship with staff will help you get a positive response.

> The attendings always knew exactly what was supposed to be done when Christine was treated for cancer, but the fellows made quite a few mistakes. I was embarrassed to correct them, but I just kept reminding myself that they had dozens of treatment plans to keep track of, and I had only one.

- Show appreciation. A short thank-you note or a plate of cookies to a doctor or nurse will be warmly received.

# Conflict resolution

Conflict is a part of life when a child's health is threatened. The heightened emotions and frequent involvement with medical bureaucracy mean that conflicts can arise easily. Because clashes are common, resolving them is crucial.

- Recognize that speaking up is difficult, especially if being assertive is uncomfortable for you. But it is very important to solve problems before they grow and interfere with a good relationship.

- Be specific and nonconfrontational when describing problems. For example, "My son gets very nervous the longer we wait for our appointment. We have waited over two hours for our last two appointments. Could we call ahead next time to see if the doctor is on schedule?" rather than, "Do you think your time is more valuable than mine?"

- Use "I" statements. For example, "I feel upset when you won't answer my questions," rather than, "You never listen to me."

- Assume mistakes will happen— only vigilance will prevent them. Try to be tactful when you point out errors.

> My two children, Sean and Angie, have had many hospitalizations for minor injuries (stitches and casts) and major procedures (benign tumor removed from chest, abdominal surgery). I have taught them to be pleasant but firm in their dealings with staff. They are good at saying, "Excuse me, but we need to wait until my mom gets here," or, "No, I don't want that done now." I have taught them that they are in charge of their own bodies. I'm proud to say that although they are never mean or threatening, they have learned to express themselves with clarity and firmness.

- Ask a hospital social worker or psychologist for advice on problem solving. Their job includes serving as mediators between staff and parents.

- Monitor your own feelings of anger and fear. Be careful not to dump on staff inappropriately. But do not let a physician or nurse behave unprofessionally toward you or your child.

- Teach your child to speak her mind. If you need to leave the room briefly, make sure you have coached your child on what to expect while you are gone.

- Do not fear reprisal for speaking up. You can be assertive without aggression.

> *I wanted to stay with Meara when she had her stitches, but the doctor was concerned that I was going to faint. So I said, "Is there anything I can do to make you more comfortable about me staying with her?" He asked, "Can you sit in a chair?" I said, "Of course." He heard what I needed, and we negotiated an agreeable solution. I sat on a chair holding my daughter's hand, and he stitched her up without worrying that I was going to fall flat on the ground.*

# CHAPTER SEVEN

# Common Procedures

*What do we live for if it is not to make
life less difficult for each other?*

—George Eliot

IF YOUR CHILD IS IN THE HOSPITAL for an emergency or a very short stay, hospital staff will handle most medical procedures. But you may be able to cajole your child into taking pills or holding still while a doctor looks in his ears better than any staff person. In the following sections, parents share techniques for helping children cope with common procedures.

## Taking pills

If your child needs regular doses of oral medication, it probably will be much easier if you try to get off to a good start and establish cooperation early. You can experiment with different techniques to find what works best for your child.

- Taste each medication. If it tastes all right, tell your child. Many pills can be chewed or swallowed whole without taste problems.

- If a medication tastes bad, you can ask your pharmacist about Flavor-X flavorings she can mix with the medication (for information about Flavor-X, call 1-800-884-5771).

*Carrie Beth was two when she became ill. She hated the taste of the pills, so I would submerge them in teaspoonfuls of pure maple syrup. The next year when she just decided she didn't want to cooperate about taking pills, I'd say to her and her two older sisters, "Strawberry gum for everybody as soon as Carrie Beth finishes her pills." Then I would leave, and the older kids encouraged her to swallow the pills.*

These are made from ordinary food flavorings and come in many flavors that kids like, including cherry and fruit punch.

Or you can ask a nurse or doctor for gel caps and pack pills inside (break them up if necessary). Gel caps come in many sizes. Number 4s are small enough for a three- or four-year-old to swallow. They are useful for any medication that bothers your child.

- Give your child a choice of drinks to accompany a pill or gel cap.

- Allow your child to chew up other food, such as chocolate chips, with medication.

- Make a game out of swallowing bad-tasting medications by having your child make the ickiest face possible as the medicine goes down. Parents also can taste the medicine and make faces.

- Give your child choices, such as, "Do you want the white pill or the six yellow pills first?"

- Crush pills in a small amount of pudding, applesauce, jam, frozen juice concentrate, or other favorite food. This is especially effective with smaller children.

- Let your child experiment with ways to administer medication, such as through a syringe. If you try this, make sure you stick to the correct dosage.

Children usually associate taking medicine with being sick, so you may have to explain why they must continue taking pills even if they feel well. Some parents say, "The pills are needed to gobble up the last few germs." Others explain that medicine can prevent the illness from returning.

*I think it's a delicate balancing act to allow a teen to be responsible for taking his own meds and yet keep some supervision of the process. Joel's meds are kept in a small basket on the kitchen counter. All meds are taken there. I'd never want him to keep his meds in his room where I would have no idea if he had taken them or not. If he had shown any resistance, I'd be doing this differently. But he's aware of the importance of each dose and the importance of his participation.*

Teenagers face different issues than small children when taking pills. Problems with teens revolve around autonomy, control, and feelings of invulnerability. Many teenagers benefit from playing an active role in their own recovery and are responsible enough to take their medication. When this is not the case, the physician, nurse, or social worker may be able to reason a resistant teenager into compliance.

Giving children all required medications is very important. Many studies show the dangers of not finishing all medications, such as the illness returning or the evolution of drug-resistant infections.

# Taking a temperature

Fever is a rise in body temperature and can be a sign of infection or disease. Fever can cause weakness, exhaustion, and dehydration.

There are several ways to take temperatures: under the tongue, under the arm, or in the ear using a special type of thermometer. Before using a rectal thermometer, check with your doctor. In some cases, they are not recommended due to the risk of tearing of tissue and infection.

- Digital thermometers can be purchased at any drug store. Some have an alarm that beeps when it is time to remove the thermometer.

- Heat-sensitive paper strips are available at drug stores or pharmacies. Dots on a temperature scale change color according to the child's temperature. They are inexpensive, and popular with many young children, however, they can be inaccurate.

- Tympanic, or ear, thermometers measure infrared waves and are very easy to use, but are expensive.

*After six-year-old Kurt's hydrocele surgery, I had to take his temperature frequently for several days. He absolutely refused to have a thermometer in his mouth. It was just impossible, so we compromised and used a digital thermometer under his arm. He complied because he liked to hear the beep at the end.*

These require proper technique to be accurate, so keep the directions handy.

Before your child leaves the hospital, ask your doctor whether you should monitor her for fever. Some fever medicines, including aspirin, can interfere with other drugs or cause complications. Find out from your doctor whether you should give medication for fever and how high the fever can go before you call.

# X-rays

Few children grow up without having x-rays to check for a broken bone or look for cavities in teeth. X-rays and imaging devices such as MRIs (magnetic resonance imaging) are important diagnostic tools.

If your child needs an x-ray, ask the technician to explain it thoroughly before you proceed. After the explanation, the technician will position your child on an x-ray table with the machine angled over him to get the best view. For a chest x-ray, your child will be strapped in a seated position.

*My four-year-old daughter needed sinus x-rays. I asked the technician to shield her chest and thyroid, but they didn't have a shield her size. So we went to another lab and they also didn't have a child-sized shield. When the technician there tried to minimize my concerns by comparing x-rays to radiation exposure from a television, I told her that I was a radiation therapist and I knew better. So, we ended up having the technician stay in the room, holding the adult shield in front of Claire's thyroid and chest, while the x-ray was taken.*

Positioning an injured limb can sometimes be painful. Most technicians try to minimize the pain, but you may have to explain to your child that he may be uncomfortable for a few moments while the technician positions his broken limb. MRIs and x-rays of internal organs are not painful.

The technician will place a heavy lead apron over the rest of the child's body to avoid exposure to radiation. Although a patient receives a small dose of radiation with each x-ray, the effects are cumulative and doctors try to expose patients to as few x-rays as possible.

When your child is in place, the technician will leave the room and will ask you to do the same. If your child is very young, the technician may give you a shield so that you can stay in the room, but this only happens when your child is unlikely to remain still on her own.

Parents and technicians usually can watch the child through a window and often there is a two-way intercom. Explaining the window and intercom can help your child stay calm.

Some children enjoy looking at their x-rays. If your child shows an interest, ask whether the doctor or technician can display the x-rays and give an explanation—it's a fun chance for your child to look at his insides.

# Casts

Casts keep broken bones immobile until they mend. They now are lighter and more manageable than the old-fashioned white plaster casts. Doctors may even give your child a choice of colors for his cast.

If your child must use a sling with the cast, you should ask for a demonstration on how to use it. Before you leave, you'll be given any special instructions, including whether the cast needs to be kept dry, how long

*Eight-year-old Sean broke his arm horribly while playing. We took him to a local orthopedic surgeon, who put on a plaster cast from wrist to armpit. It needed to be elevated at night, so we rigged up an apparatus above the couch, and Sean slept there. They put on a lightweight blue cast after the first month, followed by a bright yellow one. His friends wrote all over them. Sean was nervous about the big round saw that they used to remove the casts. I told him that he would feel some pressure, and some tickling, but no pain. We sang songs as they removed each cast.*

your child must use crutches, and when to return to have the limb checked. If your child is old enough, he'll probably appreciate being included in the discussion on taking care of the cast.

You also might ask how the doctor plans to remove the cast. Often doctors use a small saw that is noisy and may frighten your child. Ask for a demonstration to put your child's fears to rest.

# Stitches

Stitches are becoming less common for some injuries and surgeries as new options become available, including staples, butterfly bandages, and skin adhesive. You might consider whether to bring in a plastic surgeon if your child needs stitches on his face or if he could lose some function, such as from a hand injury. Unless the situation is life-threatening, there is plenty of time to discuss options.

> Sean was worried about having his stitches removed. So I got some fabric and thread and put in some stitches. I showed him with scissors how the doctor could cut the stitch and not hurt the fabric. He felt fine about it after my demonstration.

As with any medical procedure, you should get written instructions for care of stitches. Instructions might include keeping the stitches dry and measures to keep the wound from becoming infected.

# Starting an IV

Most pediatric hospitals have teams of technicians who specialize in starting IVs and drawing blood. They are usually extremely good at their jobs. An IV technician will generally use a vein in the lower arm or hand. First, the technician puts a constricting band above the site to make the veins larger and easier to see and feel. The technician then finds the vein, cleans the area, and inserts the needle. Sometimes a needle is left in place and sometimes it is removed, leaving only a thin, plastic tube in the vein. The technician makes sure the needle (or tube) is in the proper place, then covers the site with a clear dressing, and secures it with tape.

Some ways parents can help:

- Keep your child calm. The body reacts to fear by constricting the blood vessels near the skin surface. The calmer the child is, the larger his veins will be. Small children are usually calmest with a parent present; teenagers may or may not desire privacy. Listening to music, visualizing a tranquil scene (mountains covered with snow, floating in a pool), or using the same technician each time helps some children.

- Keep your child warm. Cold temperatures also cause the surface blood vessels to constrict. Wrapping the child in a blanket and putting a hot water bottle on the arm can enlarge the veins.

> *When my friends' four-year-old son was very sick, they asked me to bring him a bag of gift-wrapped things. I went to the dollar store and bought a whole bunch of little gifts and wrapped each one. They were things that he could carry into the exam room. Every time the doctor did a needle poke for blood work, he was allowed to open a gift. He loved the four tiny plastic frogs.*

- Encourage your child to drink lots of fluids. Hydration increases the fluid in the veins and makes them easier to find.

- Let gravity help. If your child is lying in bed, have her hang her arm over the side to increase the size of the vessels in the arm and hand.

- Give your child choices. If your child has a preference, let him pick the arm to be stuck. If your child is a veteran of many IVs, let him point out the best vein.

- Tell your child that it's okay to say ouch, squeeze your hand hard, or cry.

- Stop if problems develop. The secret to treating children is to spend lots of time on preparation and very little time on procedures. If a conflict arises between your child and the technician, side with your child. It's far better to take a time-out and regroup than to force the issue and lose your child's trust. Children can be remarkably cooperative if doctors and parents respect their needs and listen to their wishes.

If your child needs long-term treatments that include many needle sticks, ask about EMLA, an anesthetic cream available by prescription. EMLA is applied to the skin, covered with an airtight bandage, and left on for an hour to anesthetize the skin and underlying tissue. In some cases, it can constrict veins, so you may need to experiment to see if it works for your child.

The advice for starting an IV also applies to drawing blood from the arm. Blood is usually drawn from the large vein on the inside of the elbow using a procedure similar to starting an IV, except that the needle is removed rather than left in the arm.

> *David was poked many, many times one night and the technician could not get an IV in. We told him to stop. We said, "This child is totally blue from screaming. He's worn out." In the morning we asked the staff for the person who never misses. They brought her in and she got it on the first try.*

## Conducting tests

You may be able to save your child some discomfort by avoiding unnecessary tests. When your doctor proposes a test, the following are some questions you might ask before giving your consent.

- What is the purpose of the test?

- Does my insurance cover it?

- How will it contribute to diagnosis or treatment?

- What are the risks associated with this test?

- Are there simpler or less risky ways to get the same information?

- What are the possible side effects and how often do they occur?

- Why is it necessary to do this test now? Could we watch the symptoms and postpone the test?

- Who will do the test? Is he qualified? How many times has he done this test?

- How long will it take?

- Please explain in detail exactly what will be done during the test.

- When will the results be available?

- Are there special instructions to follow before or after the test?

- Are there any symptoms that I should call you about (such as pain, bleeding, or fatigue)?

Many tests can be done at a lab before your child is admitted to the hospital. The costs can be significantly lower. Ensure that the results of all tests done before hospitalization are sent to the hospital to prevent the need for repeated testing.

*My seven-year-old daughter needed an EEG. I asked the technician many pointed questions: What kind of room would she be in? Would other kids be there? Would she be on a bed or bench? Could I stay with her? How many electrodes would be attached to her head, and how would this be done? Would they need to shave any hair? How long does it last? Are there scary or painful parts? Is the machine loud or quiet? After I shared this information with my daughter and answered her questions, the procedure went well. I ended up getting up on the table and lying down next to her to provide some comfort.*

# CHAPTER EIGHT

# Surgery

*Next to excellence is the appreciation of it.*

—*William Makepeace Thackeray*

AS WITH MOST MEDICAL PROCEDURES, you can do a great deal to make surgery easier for your child. Preparation and communication are crucial.

## Educating yourself

When your doctor recommends surgery for your child, you should try to ensure that surgery is necessary and the surgeon is the best available. In some emergencies, you won't have time to research a surgical procedure or to meet the surgeon. But usually you will have time to find the doctor and hospital that can best help your child.

You should learn about the proposed surgical procedure and ask enough questions to thoroughly understand it. Books, the Internet, and technical articles are good places to start your search. Verify any information you obtain—some sources are thinly disguised sales pitches. Your child's doctor may also provide a video or book that explains the surgery. Ask the doctor if his technique varies from that described in these materials, so that you and your child will know what to expect.

After reading about the procedure, you will probably have a list of questions to ask your child's doctor. It helps to write questions down so you do not forget any. Either tape record or write down the doctor's answers so you can review them later.

Some parents recommend checking out the entire surgical team, especially the surgeon and anesthesiologist.

- Ask the surgeon about his qualifications and the number of times he has performed the surgery your child requires.

- Ask the surgeon what her success rate is for the surgery your child requires and how she defines success.

- Make sure the anesthesiologist is board-certified and experienced in pediatric cases.

You can also collect information through informal channels: friends in the medical field, hospital staff you've befriended, or other patients. These inquiries may seem nosy, but gathering information helps you to get the best possible care for your child.

You have the right to ask for a specific surgeon and anesthesiologist, although in some cases your insurance company may restrict your choices. Sometimes you may have to insist and/or schedule the surgery when the preferred doctor or anesthesiologist is on duty.

> We had a bad experience with an anesthesiologist and decided that from then on, we would choose our own, rather than be assigned one. I wanted someone competent and compassionate, who would talk to my teenage daughter and answer her questions. She has frequent surgeries, and I do everything I can to make it bearable.

> I asked staff at the hospital, our primary doctor, and several nurse friends for recommendations. We went to meet the doctor who received the most endorsements, and she's fabulous. We make sure the office always schedules us with Dr. V. and we call the OR the day before to confirm it was done.

## Educating your child

Most children cope best with surgery if you start preparing them as soon as you know it will take place. Explain why the surgery is necessary and what it entails. Read books about hospitals together to give your child a chance to ask questions.

You should check your child's understanding of the procedure; misunderstandings can make a child fearful. Your child likely will have questions about surgery that might not occur to you.

You also should explain anesthesia: your child will go to sleep for a short time and, when she wakes up, the surgery will be over. Young children need to understand that sleep under anesthesia is not the same as regular sleep. Explain that he will not wake up during surgery and will not remember what happens.

Try to arrange a meeting between your child and members of the medical team, particularly the surgeon and anesthesiologist. The doctors and nurses on the team can answer questions and are less likely to frighten your child if their faces are familiar.

Although I was 15 at diagnosis, I was treated at a children's hospital. The food was kid-oriented, the staff were mostly very calm ("So you wanna go downstairs and see the goldfish? No problem!"), and here's the part I thought was really sweet: You can take your favorite stuffed toys to surgery with you. I took my teddy bear -he's been with me since I was a couple of weeks old, and is kind of raggedy but still cute— and my two favorite Bibles to both my surgeries. They didn't move them until I was completely "out" and put them back when they transferred me to recovery, so I never missed them at all.

Your child also needs to know that he will ride to surgery in a bed on wheels and, in the operating room, doctors and nurses will wear blue face masks and hair nets and outfits that look like blue pajamas. You can tell your child that, even though he has met the surgeon, it's sometimes hard to identify her among the other blue-masked people.

Your doctor or surgeon can explain to your child what to expect after surgery: an IV, catheter, bandages, stitches, scars, or the need for crutches or a wheelchair. Also, try to prepare your child for any pain. For example, her throat will hurt after her tonsils are removed or his belly may ache after an appendectomy. Most children can tolerate some discomfort, but they do better when prepared for it.

People who have undergone the surgery before can answer many of your child's questions. And, even with minor surgeries, children often wonder whether they might die. Meeting people who have survived a surgery intact can be a great comfort.

Other information to obtain prior to surgery:

- Instructions for the night before. Find out if there are any prohibitions against eating and drinking. Scheduling the surgery for early morning can prevent hunger and thirst from becoming a problem.

*My daughter, Claire, has been hospitalized twice, for a tonsillectomy and to have tubes put in her ears. Before both surgeries, we took her to the grocery store to pick out popsicles and ice cream for when she came home. We went to the bookstore where she picked books to read and the movie rental store for movies. We also let her choose new sheets for her bed and new pajamas. All these things gave her some control over what was going to happen, as well as something exciting to look forward to after the surgery. It allowed us to explain that she would be sore and tired, but we could still have a fun time.*

- Prescriptions. If you can get prescriptions for medications ahead of time, it may be far easier on you to fill them before the surgery, rather than after.

- Ask whether there will be any restrictions on diet or exercise after the surgery.

# The surgery

Some hospitals allow parents to be present when a child is anesthetized, others don't. Many parents feel strongly that they should be present until their child is safely sedated. Some have changed hospitals or won a temporary change in hospital procedure in order to stay with their child.

Your child may be frightened when an anesthesia mask is placed over his face. Many anesthesiologists will give the child a choice of gas flavorings to make the mask more acceptable. If you are present, you can comfort your child by holding his hand, singing to him, telling stories, or simply making sure he can see you until he falls asleep.

Much as you'd like to, you cannot follow your child into surgery. The wait may be difficult, but this is a good time to get a breath of fresh air, eat something, make a telephone call, or take a quick break from hospital routine. Your child will need you when she wakes up and the more relaxed and comfortable you are, the better both you and your child will feel.

# The recovery room

Some hospitals allow parents into the recovery room, others do not. Find out the hospital's policy and explain this to your child prior to surgery so your child will know what to expect upon awakening.

Whether you meet your child in the recovery room or later, comfort him

> I told the staff that I needed to be with Christine when she was anesthetized and when she woke up. Going into the recovery room was not standard practice, so the surgeon made the arrangements well before the surgery. When they gave Christine the pre-op meds, she got very goofy and giggly. She smiled and waved to me as they pushed her gurney into the OR. After the surgery, I was the first thing she saw when she opened her eyes.

any way you can: hold his hand, rock him, sing songs, play music, watch TV, or read him a book.

# Coming home

You may have to provide some medical care when your child comes home. If so, arrange to have the necessary medical equipment at home before your child leaves the hospital. Also try to make any special accommodations in advance, such as creating a sleeping area downstairs if your child cannot manage the stairs. If your hospital has a discharge planner or social worker, talk with her well before your child's discharge time, to make sure that you have all the information you need.

If your child needs nursing care, physical therapy, or other services after she leaves the hospital, make sure the doctor states that in the discharge papers. Some insurers refuse to pay for care after hospitalization unless there is a documented medical need.

Your family may need a few days or weeks to rest and recover before life returns to normal. Don't be afraid to tell family and friends that you need some down time for a few days after your child comes home. Hospitalization can be very stressful for families and everyone may benefit from time to decompress.

*After Claire had her tonsillectomy, she was feeling pretty good. A friend and her three children came to visit her at home that evening. The kids went out and played hard: swinging on the swings and running around. I should have known to keep her calmer and told them to go home much earlier. The visit really stressed her system and she was very ill for the next two days.*

# CHAPTER NINE

# Pain Management

*Pain is a thing that is glad to be forgotten.*

*—Robinson Jeffers*

MOST HOSPITALIZATIONS RESULT IN SOME degree of pain for children. Procedures such as blood draws, IV insertions, setting a bone, or getting stitches are common, painful events. The first few days after surgery usually are also painful.

Great strides have been made in identifying and treating pediatric pain. The two primary methods to prevent pain caused by procedures are psychological (using the mind) and pharmacological (using drugs).

## Psychological method

There is no fear greater than fear of the unknown. If children understand what is going to happen, where it will happen, who will be there, and what it will feel like, they will be better able to cope. Ask the hospital's child life specialist, psychologist, or trained nurse to discuss and practice different methods of pain management with your child.

*Seven-year-old Tayler needed frequent blood draws to monitor her dilantin [medication for seizures] levels. Before the first one, we bought a new doll and poked her with needles. Then we went to the lab and met Barb— the technician. She told Tayler about her dogs (their pictures were on the walls). They really connected. Barb showed her the needles and let Tayler watch some people have their blood drawn. Barb reassured her that, "I am very good and very fast at this." Tayler felt much better after the visit.*

- Explain each step in the procedure. Even if you think the child understands, ask him to tell you what he thinks will happen. Many parents are very surprised by their child's misconceptions.

- If possible, meet the person who will perform the procedure and let your child ask questions.

- Tour the room where the procedure will take place.

- See the instruments that will be used.

- Allow small children to play the procedure with dolls.

- Let older children observe a demonstration on a doll.

- Show adolescents videotapes that describe the procedure.

- Encourage discussion and answer all questions.

*I discovered my special place when I was 12, during a relaxation session. My place is surrounded by sand and tall, fanning palm trees are everywhere. The sky is always clear; the sun shines bright. Each time I come to this place I lie down to feel the gritty sand beneath me. Once in awhile I get up and go looking for seashells. I feel the breeze going right through me, and I can smell the salt water. Whenever I feel sad or alone, or if I am in pain, I usually go jump in the water because it is a soothing place for me. I like to float in the water because it gives me a refreshing feeling that nobody can hurt me there.*

There's no substitute for good preparation to help your child get through a medical procedure. But you may also be able to use psychological techniques to lessen your child's pain.

- Hypnosis is a well-documented method for reducing discomfort during painful procedures. Hypnosis requires individualized treatment for each child, so it must be available at your child's hospital or you will need to locate a private practitioner.

- Parents can teach imagery, which is similar to hypnosis. Children must practice imagery techniques before the procedure. Have your child visually focus on one object in the room, hold your hand, breathe deeply, and imagine a tranquil scene. (Some sources of information about these techniques are listed in the Resources section of this book.)

- You can use distraction techniques with all age groups, but it should not be used as a substitute for preparation. Colorful, moving objects will distract babies. Parents can distract preschoolers by showing picture books or videos, telling stories, singing songs, or blowing bubbles. Hugging a favorite stuffed animal comforts many youngsters. School-age children and teens can watch videos or television, or listen to music. Several institutions use interactive videos to help distract older children or teens.

- Many stores and hospital resource rooms carry relaxation or visualization tapes that children can listen to using headphones.

Other therapies that are used successfully to help deal with medical treatments are relaxation, biofeedback, massage, and acupuncture.

# Pharmacological method

Some hospitals offer sedation or anesthesia for painful procedures; others do not. Sometimes anesthesia is available only for infants or overwhelmingly anxious children. If painful procedures distress your child, explore all available options for pain relief.

The ideal pain relief drug for children should be easy to administer, have minimal and predictable effects, provide adequate pain relief, and last for a

*Ten-year-old Sean fell and cut his forehead down to the bone. I took him to the emergency room and told them that he scars easily and we needed a plastic surgeon to do the repair. They resisted; I insisted. We ended up waiting four hours. The plastic surgeon sprayed on an anesthetic then waited a few minutes before giving the shots of anesthetic. Sean didn't feel a thing, which was good because it required many internal and surface stitches. The scar is now so faint that you don't notice it.*

short time. Pain medication for procedures can be given by IV, on the skin, by mouth, and occasionally by lollipop.

There are many types of drugs and several methods used to administer them. Procedures can be done with local anesthetic, temporary sedation, or general anesthesia. Discuss with your doctor and anesthesiologist which method will work best for your child.

All sedation can result in complications, the most common is slowing or cessation of breathing. Trained, experienced personnel should handle the sedation and your child should be monitored until she recovers fully.

# Determining if your child is in pain

Infants, toddlers, school-aged children, and teenagers all show pain in different ways.

*My son was in pediatric intensive care with a fractured skull from a bike accident. They had him sedated but I didn't think they were giving him adequate pain medication. He was unconscious but still crying. The nurse called the doctor but couldn't get the instructions changed. I asked her to note on the chart, "Parent demands to meet with doctor first thing in the morning to discuss pain management."*

*In the morning, in walked a new doctor (the first had gone on vacation) who said, "Hello, my name is Dr. S., I have rewritten the orders to eliminate the sedation and increase his pain meds." Problem solved.*

- Infants in pain move less. They may become irritable and cry frequently. Their appetites decrease. They may cry out if moved or touched. Parents know their infants well, and should advocate for appropriate medication if their infant is in pain.

- Toddlers may become irritable, cry, or strike out if they are in pain. They may lose all interest in playing. Their breathing can become rapid and shallow. They might not be able to describe the pain in words, but may point to what hurts if asked, "Where is your owie?"

- School-aged children will be able to tell you when they are hurting. You can ask your child where it hurts, and how much. Nurses should have sheets with a series of faces (from smiling to crying) that may help your child explain the amount of pain he is feeling. Some young children won't express pain because they fear that they will "get a shot." Take time beforehand to explain that they can get pain medicine through an IV line or by mouth and that the medicine will make them feel better, not worse.

- Teenagers react to pain like adults do. They may become angry, withdraw, have disrupted sleep and appetites, or become quiet and still. Any behavior changes should be investigated. Teens frequently don't report pain for fear of taking drugs or becoming addicted. Reassure your teen that patients rarely become addicted to pain medication. Once the pain subsides, it is easy to stop taking the medications. Accurate, factual information about pain and pain control are crucial for adolescents.

## Medications used to treat pain

Children's pain is typically treated with the same drugs used for adults. Mild pain may be treated with acetaminophen (Tylenol). Mild narcotics, such as codeine, are used for moderate pain. Severe pain—such as might be experienced the first few days after major surgery—can be effectively treated with a wide range of medications. These drugs can be given by mouth, by IV, in a suppository, or by injection (rare in children).

Taking pain medication will prevent your child's pain from becoming unbearable. Adhere closely to the physician's directions to keep a constant level of medication in your child's body. If you wait until your child is in pain before giving the medication, it will take a greater dose for your child to become comfortable again.

If the prescribed drugs are not curbing your child's pain, or your child is very nauseated, tell the nurse and doctor. Most hospitals have a "pain team" of specialists in pain control. Ask for a consultation with this team if the staff cannot manage your child's pain or nausea.

# CHAPTER TEN

# Family and Friends: What to Say

*Shared joy is double joy, shared sorrow is half sorrow.*

—*Swedish proverb*

AN ILLNESS OR INJURY SERIOUS ENOUGH to require hospitalization creates a ripple effect, first touching the immediate family, then extended family, friends, coworkers, schoolmates, church members, and the entire community. Families can experience loving support and generous help, as well as disappointment. Parents will find family and friends who help them in extraordinary ways. But sometimes, those who could provide the greatest support may become sources of added stress.

## Notifying family and friends

If your child goes to the hospital for a routine procedure or minor injury, you probably won't have to communicate with anyone outside the immediate family. When the illness or injury is serious, notifying family and friends becomes a painful necessity.

The easiest way to tell family and friends is to delegate one person to do the job. Calling one relative, neighbor, or close friend prevents numerous conversations about the illness or injury. Most parents are at their child's bedside and want to avoid more emotional upheaval, especially in front of their child. Parents need to recognize that relatives' and friends' emotions will mirror their own: shock, fear, worry, helplessness. Since most loved ones want to help but don't know what to do or say, they welcome cues about what might help.

# Communication

Families need to clearly communicate what will help. A telephone chain is a good way to keep family and friends informed of your child's progress. Or you can delegate a family member as communicator. This person will relay information to another person, who then telephones another. Some families also leave updates on their telephone answering machines.

Sometimes, especially when an illness or injury is severe, parents must take extra steps to keep family members and friends informed and involved.

- Encourage all members of the family to keep in touch through visits, calls, mail, videotapes, cassette tapes, or pictures.

- Call if you don't hear from family members or close friends. Often silence means they don't know what to do or say.

- Tell family members and friends when your child is too sick or too fatigued for company. When visits are welcome, make them brief and cheerful. Long visits can distress sick children and overtax tired parents.

*The first three days in the hospital I spent much of my time crying on the phone when talking to friends and relatives. Then I realized how frightening this must be to my two-year-old. So I just took the phone off the hook and left it there. Now, each time Jennifer is hospitalized, I call one friend and have her spread the news, then I take the phone off the hook again and concentrate on my daughter.*

# What to say

Many people feel awkward and tongue-tied in the presence of families with an injured or ill child, particularly if the injury or illness is severe. Kind words are always welcome and a specific offer of help can be accepted or graciously declined.

- I am so sorry.

- I didn't call earlier because I didn't know what to say.

- Our family would like to do your yard work. We will mow the lawn, weed the flower beds, and rake the leaves.

- We want to clean your house for you once a week. What day would be convenient?

- Would it help if we took care of your dog (or cat, or bird)? We would love to do it.

- I walk my dog three times a day. May I walk yours, too?

- The church is setting up a system to deliver meals to your house. When is the best time to drop them off?

- I will take care of your children whenever you need to take Jimmy to the hospital. Call us any time, day or night, and we will come pick them up.

# Things that do not help

Out of ignorance, people sometimes say hurtful things to parents of sick or injured children. If you are a family member or friend of a parent with a hospitalized child, please do not say any of the following:

- "God only gives people what they can handle." Some people cannot handle the stress related to their child's illness or injury.

- "I know just how you feel." Unless you have a child in a similar situation, you simply don't know.

- "You are so brave," or, "You are so strong." Parents of very sick children are not heroes; they are ordinary people struggling with extraordinary stress.

Parents also make the following suggestions of things to avoid doing:

> Many well-wishing friends always said, "Let me know what I can do." I wish they had just "done," instead of asking for direction. It took too much energy to decide, call them, and make arrangements. I wish someone would have said, "When is your clinic day? I'll bring dinner," or, "I'll baby-sit Sunday afternoon so you and your husband can go out to lunch together."

- Do not say, "Let us know if there is anything we can do." It is far better to make a specific suggestion.

- Do not make personal comments in front of the child: "He's lost so much weight," or, "She's so pale."

- Do not do things that require the parent to support you (for example, call up repeatedly, crying).

- Especially if treatments are lengthy, do not talk continually about the illness. Some normal conversations are welcome.

- Do not ask "What if" questions: What if he can't go to school? What if your insurance won't cover it? What if she gets sicker? Parents only can deal with the present.

Most parents welcome stories of other children you know who had a similar condition and are doing fine. Do not share stories about children who are not doing well, who have long-term side effects, or who have died.

# Serious illness: Losing friends

Serious illnesses, such as childhood cancer, or serious injuries, such as damage to the spinal cord or brain, put tremendous strain on everyone. Unfortunately, most parents of children with a long-term illness or permanent injury lose friends. Some friends can't cope and either suddenly disappear, or gradually fade away. Often, you can keep a friend by staying in touch, but sometimes, they just can't handle the stress.

Some parents distribute newsletters to their friends describing their child's progress and the stress the family is under. The newsletter gives friends an option: they can stay in touch or tune out.

> *He was in and out of the hospital for three years and, except for one good friend, none of my friends called when I was home. It seemed that after the initial three-month crisis, they removed themselves from the situation, as often happens.*

# CHAPTER ELEVEN

# Family and Friends: How to Help

*We can do no great things—only small things with great love.*

—*Mother Theresa*

A CHILD'S SERIOUS SICKNESS OR INJURY can overwhelm a family—straining time, finances, and emotions. Help from friends and relatives is a crucial part of the family's ability to cope with the disruption in their lives.

Many relatives and friends genuinely want to help, but don't know how. The following sections describe helpful things you can do for a family with a child in the hospital. Although some of the suggestions listed are most appropriate when dealing with lengthy illnesses or recoveries, they may give you some good ideas for any hospitalization.

## Help at the hospital

Friends and family members can find many ways to make a child's hospital experience more enjoyable.

- Send balloon bouquets, funny cards, posters, toys, or humorous books. A cheerful hospital room really boosts a child's spirits.

- Send funny videotapes or arrive with a good joke. Laughter helps heal the mind and body.

*One of the nicest things that friends did was to bring a huge picnic basket full of food to the hospital. We spread a blanket on the floor, Erica crawled out of bed, and the entire family sat down together and ate. Most people don't realize how expensive it is to have to eat every meal at the hospital cafeteria, so the picnic was not only fun, but helped us save a few dollars.*

- Bring toys. Puzzles, games, picture books, coloring books, age-appropriate computer games (you could supply a portable computer if the child doesn't have one available), CDs or tapes, and crafts are welcome.

- Bring a basket of snacks and juice for family members.

- Offer to give parents a break from the hospital room. A walk outside, shopping trip, haircut, or a long shower can be very refreshing.

- Donate frequent flyer miles to distant family members who have the time—but not the money—to help, if the treatment or illness is lengthy or severe.

# Household

Parents of sick or injured children often cannot handle day-to-day chores. Friends and family can help with these routine tasks. Even when the illness or injury is not too severe, a home-cooked meal or a bag of small toys can express love and provide comfort.

- Provide meals.

- Take care of pets or livestock.

- Mow grass, shovel snow, rake leaves, weed gardens.

- Clean house.

- Grocery shop (especially when the family is due home from the hospital).

- Do laundry. Drop off and pick up dry cleaning.

- Provide a place to stay near the hospital.

> *Friends from home sent boxes of art supplies to us when the whole family spent those first ten weeks in the Ronald McDonald House far from home. They sent scissors, paints, paper, colored pens. It was a great help for Carrie Beth and her two sisters. One friend even sent an Easter package with straw hats for each girl, and flowers, ribbons, and glue to decorate them with.*

# Siblings

Siblings of hospitalized children need lots of love, attention, and care. Friends and family can help when parents are overwhelmed.

- Baby-sit whenever parents go to doctor's appointments, the emergency room, or during a prolonged hospital stay.

- When parents are home with a sick child, take siblings to a park, sports event, or movie.

- Invite siblings over for meals.

- If you bring a gift for the sick child, bring something for the siblings.

- Offer to help siblings with homework.

- Drive siblings to lessons, games, or school.

- Listen to siblings when they need to talk.

> *My friends were supportive, rather than critical, in the months after my son was diagnosed with cancer. Parents in crisis do strange things, sometimes. I tore out my old kitchen to completely remodel it. Some people thought I was crazy, but my old friends knew I needed something to take my mind off my son's illness. Their understanding really helped.*

# Psychological support

Parents of a sick or injured child can feel overwhelmed, frightened, and exhausted. They need practical and emotional help from family and friends.

- Call frequently. Be open to listening if parents want to talk about their feelings.

- Call to talk about topics other than the child's illness or injury.

- Stay in the hospital with the sick child if parents have to work.

- Call the social worker at the local hospital to find out if there are support groups for parents and/or kids in your area if you think the family might be interested.

- Drive parent and child to the hospital.

- Buy books (humorous or uplifting ones) for family members if they are readers.

- Send cards, letters, faxes, audio cassettes, or videotapes.

- Baby-sit the sick child so parents can go out to eat, exercise, take a walk, or just get out of the hospital.

- Donate blood. Your blood won't necessarily be used for the injured child, but will replenish the general supply.

- Give lots of hugs.

> Word got around my parents' hometown, and I received cards from many high school acquaintances, who still cared enough to call or write and say we're praying for you, please let us know how things are going. It was so neat to get so many cards out of the blue that said, "I'm thinking about you."

## Financial support

Helping a family keep track of finances while a child is sick or injured can be a great gift. Even fully insured families can spend up to twenty-five percent of their income on copayments, travel, motels, meals, and other uncovered items when a child has a long-term, serious illness or injury. Uninsured or underinsured families can lose their savings, or even their house. Friends and family can find many ways to help.

- Start a support fund. (Refer to *A Special Way to Care*, by Sheila Peterson, listed in the Resources section.)

- Share leave. The federal government and some companies have leave banks that permit people who are ill or taking care of someone who is ill to use coworkers' leave so they won't lose pay.

> My husband's coworkers didn't collect money, they did something even more valuable. They donated sick leave hours, so that he was able to be at the hospital frequently during those first few months without losing a paycheck.

- Job share. Some families work out job-share arrangements in which a coworker donates time to perform part of a job to enable a parent to spend time at the hospital. Job sharing allows the job to get done, keeps peace at work, and prevents financial losses for the family. Friends with similar skills (word processing, filing, or sales, for example) might be allowed to rotate through the job on a volunteer basis to cover for an ill child's parent.

- Collect money by organizing a bake sale, dance, or raffle.

- Give the family gift certificates from restaurants that deliver meals.

- Handle hospital bills. Keeping track of medical bills can be time-consuming, frustrating, and exhausting. If you are a close relative or friend, you could offer to review, organize, and file (or enter into a computer) the voluminous paperwork. Making calls and writing letters about contested claims or billing errors are very helpful.

# Help from schoolmates

Classmates and friends can be a huge help to a sick or injured child by giving him support and encouragement and helping him feel that he hasn't lost touch.

*Brent's kindergarten class sent a packet containing a picture drawn for him by each child in the class. They also made him a book. Another time they sent him a letter written on huge poster board. He couldn't wait to get back to school.*

- Encourage visits (if appropriate), cards, and phone calls from classmates.

- Make sure the visiting children are prepared for what they will see at the hospital. Tell their parents, "Joey will have a tube in his nose," or, "Carrie's skin will be puffy."

- Ask the teacher to send the school newspaper and other news along with assignments.

- Classmates can sign a brightly colored banner to send to the hospital.

- The teacher or principal can put the entire class on a speakerphone to chat with their classmate.

- Make a video of your child in the hospital to send to classmates. He can describe his life in the hospital, introduce the nurses and doctors, or take them on a tour. Then have the classmates send a video back. These can become treasured keepsakes.

# Religious support

Your church and religious community can be an enormous source of spiritual and practical help.

- Arrange for the pastor, rabbi, or church members to visit the hospital, if the family wants.

- Arrange prayer services for the sick child.

- Ask the child's Sunday school class (or whatever class is appropriate for the family's denomination) to send pictures, posters, letters, balloons, or tapes to the sick child.

*The day our son was diagnosed, we raced next door to ask our wonderful neighbors to take care of our dog. The news of his diagnosis quickly spread, and we found out later that five neighborhood families gathered that very night to pray for Brent.*

# CHAPTER TWELVE

# Feelings and Behavior

*Example is not the main thing in influencing others—it is the only thing.*

—Albert Schweitzer

UNDER THE BEST OF CIRCUMSTANCES, childrearing can be daunting. When parenting is complicated by a crisis, such as a serious illness, communication within the family may suffer. In normal times, children know the family rules and understand the limits on their behavior. When extremely stressful events occur, normal family life is disrupted, and confusing and distressing feelings may appear. Parenting must change in response to the shifting needs of children in crisis.

## Feelings

Children generally have fewer coping skills than adults. They can be overcome with feelings when they are sick or hurt. At varying times and to varying degrees, children and teens may feel fearful, angry, resentful, powerless, violated, lonely, weird, inferior, incompetent, betrayed. All these feelings, if left unresolved, create stress. Children need to learn ways to deal with these feelings to prevent acting out (by throwing tantrums, for example) or acting in (becoming depressed or withdrawn).

> *I have found that as my children's understanding deepens, they come back with more questions, needing more detailed answers. So, my motto is, be honest but don't scare them. If you say everything is okay but you are crying, they know something is wrong, and that they can't trust you to tell the truth.*

Good communication is the first step toward helping your family cope with the feelings and changes brought about by illness or injury.

- **Honesty**. Above all, children must be able to trust their parents. They can face almost anything when they know their parents will be at their side. Trust requires honesty. For children to feel secure, they must know they can depend on their parents to tell them the truth, be it good news or bad.

- **Listening**. When you are coping with your child's illness or injury, just getting through each day can consume most of your time, attention, and energy. So time is one of the greatest gifts you can give your children. They need a special time when you really focus on what they are saying, listen to the words, and the feelings behind them, a time when you stop to think before speaking.

- **Talking**. If you do not usually talk to your children about how you feel, it can be difficult to start in a crisis. But you can try. You can provide an opening by saying, for example, "I really miss you and feel sad when dad takes you to the hospital." Or, "The teacher called to talk about your schoolwork. I was relieved to hear her ideas on keeping up with homework. Have you been worried about school?" These conversa-

*When my daughter was seven, three years after her treatment ended, I realized how important it is to keep listening. She was complaining about a hangnail so I told her I would cut it. She yelled I would hurt her. I asked, "When have I ever hurt you?" She said, "In the hospital." I sat down and rocked her in my arms, explained what had happened in the hospital during her treatment, why we had to bring her, and how we felt about it. I asked her feelings about being there. We cleared the air that day, and I expect we will need to talk about it many more times. Then she held out her hand so that I could cut her hangnail.*

tions also create an opportunity for your child to share her feelings.

- Touching. This is a good time to give children lots of back rubs and hugs. Children, sick or well, need frequent contact with parents. Be sure your kids know you have an unlimited supply of hugs.

# Checklist for parenting stressed children

Some parents like to keep a list of reminders about how to handle children when both parties are stressed.

- Be a model of the type of behavior you desire. If you talk respectfully and take timeouts when angry, your child will learn to do likewise. If you scream and hit, that is how your child will handle his anger.

- Seek professional help for behaviors that trouble you.

- Teach your child to talk about her feelings.

- Listen to your child with understanding and empathy.

- Be honest and admit your mistakes.

- Help your child examine why she is behaving as she is.

- Distinguish between having feelings (always okay) and acting on feelings in destructive or hurtful ways (not okay).

- Have clear rules and consequences for violations.

- Discuss acceptable outlets for anger.

*At one point Caitlin had overeaten her beloved French fries and had a "worse than agony case of gas," as she described it. She spent the evening howling and really created a stir on the pediatric floor. She had a classic tantrum. I went in to take a shower and, when I returned to her room, there was a note taped to her door apologizing to all the people on the floor for her screaming attack.*

- Give frequent reassurances of your love.

- Provide lots of hugs and physical affection.

- Compliment your child for good behavior.

- Recognize that disturbing behaviors can result from stress, pain, and drugs.

- Remember that with lots of structure, love, and time, problems will become more manageable.

# Behavior changes

Some children, due to temperament and upbringing, are blessed with good coping abilities. They understand what is expected and they find ways to do it. Many parents express great admiration for their child's strength and grace in the face of adversity. Most family members, however, respond to the illness in the family with changes in feelings and behavior.

- **Anger.** Parents often respond to illness or injury with anger. So do children. Children rage at their pain and at their parents for bringing them to the hospital to be hurt more. Sick or injured children have good reasons to be angry. Encourage them to vent their feelings in appropriate ways, such as punching pillows, screaming in the back yard, or keeping a journal.

- **Problems sleeping.** Children often express stress by feeling unable to sleep alone or by having nightmares. Some parents allow the child

> Our son has a serious condition that has required years of difficult treatments. He is either very defiant or an absolute angel. Sometimes he argues about every single thing. I think it is because he has had so little control in his life. I have clear rules, am very firm, and put my foot down. But I also try to choose my battles wisely, so that we can have good times, too. My husband reminds me that if he wasn't this type of tough kid, he wouldn't have made it through the years of treatment, including so many setbacks.

to sleep with them, while others try soothing bedtime rituals or seek therapy.

- **Tantrums.** Healthy children have tantrums when they are overwhelmed by their feelings. So do sick or injured children. You often can predict tantrums by paying close attention to what triggers the outburst. This can help you prevent tantrums by avoiding situations that overload your child.

- **Withdrawal.** Some children withdraw rather than blow up in anger. Like denial, withdrawal can temporarily help a child come to grips with strong feelings. However, too much withdrawal can be a sign of depression or psychological trauma. Parents or counselors can gently encourage withdrawn children to express their feelings.

- **Regression.** Many parents worry if children regress to using a special comfort object when they are sick or hurt. Many young children return to using a bottle, or cling to a favorite toy or blanket. Allow your child to use whatever he can to find comfort. The behaviors usually stop when the child starts feeling better or when treatment ends.

> *In the first few days of hospitalization for cancer, my three-year-old daughter stopped interacting with everyone. She lay on the bed with her face turned to the wall. She wouldn't talk, make eye contact, or respond in any way. She would totally ignore us if we tried to comfort her with stories, songs, or hugs. She tuned us out. We asked for help and a psychiatric nurse worked with her for two hours. We don't know what she did, but when we came back in, our daughter was sitting up in bed painting her fingernails.*

# Communication and discipline

Short-term hospitalizations or outpatient surgeries may create only minor disruptions in your family's routines. However, long-term treatments or lengthy hospitalization increases the need for consistent rules. Parents of children with difficult or long-term illnesses share the following techniques to help improve communication and maintain discipline within the family.

- Make sure all the children clearly understand the family rules. Stressed children feel safer in homes with structured, predictable routines.

- Enforce family rules consistently. Make sure all caregivers know the rules.

> *All these interns at the teaching hospital came in and said, "Can we listen to David's heart?" He sat up and said, "You ask me." All the females got to listen and none of the males. He wanted to control who listened to his heart and he only picked the female interns.*

- Give kids some power. Offer choices and, as appropriate, let them control some aspects of their lives and medical treatment.

- Take charge of incoming gifts. Too many gifts can make an ill child worry ("If I'm getting all of these great presents, things must be really bad"). Gifts also make siblings jealous. Be specific if you want people not to bring gifts, or if you want gifts for each child, not just the sick one. When a child has an illness or injury that requires long-term care, some parents gather the gifts and hand them out at regular intervals throughout treatment.

- Find acceptable ways to physically release anger. Children can ride a bike, run around the house, swing, play basketball or soccer, pound nails into wood, mold clay, punch pillows, yell, take a shower or bath, or draw angry pictures.

- Teach your child to use words to express her anger, for example, "It makes me furious when you do that," or, "I am so mad I feel like hitting you." Releasing anger physically and expressing anger verbally are both valuable life skills to master.

- Treat the sick or hurt child as normally as possible.

- Try to determine whether the illness or injury is aggravating a preexisting problem. If so, treat the problem, not the symptoms.

- Find a professional counselor who specializes in children whenever you are concerned about your child's behavior. Mental health professionals know how to resolve problems—give them a chance to help you.

- Teach children relaxation or visualization skills to help them cope with their feelings.

- If your child likes to draw, paint, knit, do collages, or other artwork, encourage it. Art is soothing and therapeutic. It allows the child a positive outlet for feelings and creativity. Making something beautiful really helps raise children's spirits.

> *Jody was continually making "projects" when he was in the bone marrow transplant unit. We kept him supplied with a fishing box full of materials, and he glued and taped and constructed all sorts of sculptures. He did beautiful drawings full of color, and every person he drew always had hands shaped like hearts. If we asked him what he was making, he always answered, "I'll show you when I'm done."*

Allow your child to be totally in charge of his art. Do not make suggestions or criticize (by saying, "stay inside the lines," or, "skies need to be blue not orange"). Rather, encourage him and praise his efforts. Display the artwork in your home or your child's hospital room. Listen carefully if your child offers an explanation of the art, but do not pry if it is private. Being supportive will allow your child to explore ways to soothe himself and clarify his feelings.

- Help your child start and keep a journal to draw in and to record feelings, events, and visits. This can become an important emotional outlet.

- Have reasonable expectations. If you are expecting a sick four-year-old to act like a healthy six-year-old, or a teenager to act like an adult, you are setting your child up to fail.

- Give children time to process the experience of illness, hospitalization, and treatment. Many children will talk about their hospital experience or recreate it when they play for months after returning home.

# CHAPTER THIRTEEN

# Siblings

*We are all in the same boat, in a stormy sea,*
*and we owe each other a terrible loyalty.*

—*G.K. Chesterton*

A CHILD'S HOSPITALIZATION TOUCHES all members of the family, especially siblings. Even a short-term hospital stay can disrupt a sibling's sense of security and routine. An illness or injury in the family creates an array of conflicting emotions in siblings. They worry about their ill brother or sister yet resent the turmoil in their family. They often feel jealous of the gifts and attention showered on the sick child and then guilty for having these emotions.

Even parents who do not anticipate problems can benefit by knowing about the range of emotional responses that can occur and how to help siblings cope. You will be on the lookout for responses, will understand that they are normal, and can act more quickly to deal with them.

## Emotional responses

A child's illness or injury can deeply upset her brothers and sisters. If the injury is serious, or the illness pro-

> *My older daughter spent a lot of time in the hospital. Her younger sister (three years old) vacillated between fear of catching her sister's illness and wishing she was ill so that she would get the gifts and attention ("I want to get sick and go to the hospital with mommy"). She developed many fears and had frequent nightmares. We did lots of medical play which seemed to help her. I let her direct the action, using puppets or dolls, and I discovered that she thought there was lots of violence during her sister's treatments.*

longed, there is no time, and little energy, to focus on the siblings. Siblings may be flooded with anger and concern, jealousy and love. They may be in conflict as never before. Yet they often have no one to turn to for help. If you recognize that siblings' emotions are normal, not pathological, you will be better able to help your children talk about and cope with their strong feelings.

A sibling may experience a range of emotions.

- **Concern.** Children really worry about a sick brother or sister. It is hard for them to watch someone they love be hurt by an injury, surgery, or treatment. It is hard to feel so healthy and full of energy when your brother or sister has to stay in the hospital. And when an illness or injury is serious, siblings may know that death is a possibility.

- **Fear.** Even if a brother or sister is injured or suffering from a non-communicable illness, siblings often worry that they, their parents, or friends can "catch it." An illness or injury can change a child's view that the world is a safe place. Depending on their age, siblings worry that their brother or sister may get sicker. Some siblings develop symptoms of illness in an attempt to regain attention from the parents.

Fear of other things may emerge: fear of being hit by a car, fear of dogs, fear of strangers. Many worries can be quieted by accurate and age-appropriate explanations from parents or medical staff.

> *My fifteen-year-old daughter has severe endometriosis. It has required six surgeries and many ER visits. Because it's a disease that you can't see, her younger brother has a hard time accepting it. He says things like, "You're with her all the time," and, "She's just faking being sick." I realize that we need to explain the situation again and also make special time for him. We need to give him plenty of love and support, too.*

- **Jealousy.** Despite feeling concerned for an ill brother or sister, almost all siblings also feel jealous. Presents and cards flood in for the sick child, mom and dad stay at the hospital with the sick child, and most conversations revolve around the sick child. When the siblings go out to play, the neighbors ask about the sick child. At school, teachers are concerned about the sick child. Is it any wonder that they feel jealous?

- **Guilt.** Young children are egocentric; they believe the world revolves around them. It is logical for them to feel that they caused the illness or injury. They may have said in anger, "I hope you get sick and die," and then their brother got sick.

  You should try to dispel this notion. Children should be told that sickness and injury just happen, and no one in the family causes them. They need to understand that thinking something or saying something doesn't make it happen.

  Beyond feeling guilt for causing the illness or injury, most siblings feel guilt for normal responses, such as anger and jealousy. They think, "How can I feel this way about my brother when he's so sick?" Assure them that conflicting feelings are normal and expected.

- **Abandonment.** If parental attention revolves around the sick child, siblings may feel isolated and resentful. Even when parents make a con-

> *One day when my four-year-old son was in day care, we had to unexpectedly bring Erica in for emergency surgery on a septic hip. I called day care and said that I couldn't pick up Daniel by closing time. The teacher said, "No problem, I'll take him home for dinner." When we got Daniel that evening, he was very withdrawn. Later, he exclaimed, "All the mommies came. Then teacher turned out the lights, and you didn't come to get me," and he burst into tears. In hindsight, one of us should have gone to bring him to the hospital to sit with us. It was tense there, but at least he would have been with us.*

scious effort not to be preoccupied with their ill child, siblings often believe that they are not getting their fair share of attention, and may feel rejected.

- **Sadness.** Siblings have good reasons to be sad. They miss their parents and the normal routine of daily life. Some children show their sadness by crying often, others withdraw and become depressed. Many children confide in relatives or friends that they think their parents don't love them anymore.

- **Anger.** Siblings' lives are in turmoil and, being human, they feel a need to blame someone. It's natural for them to think that if their brother didn't get sick, life would be back to normal. When the illness or injury is severe, questions such as, "Why did this happen to us?" or, "Why can't things be the way they used to be?" are common. Children's anger may be directed at their sick brother, their parents, relatives, friends, or doctor. The anger may have many triggers, such as being left with baby-sitters, unequal application of family rules, or additional responsibilities at home. Because each member of the family may have frayed nerves, angry outbursts can occur.

- **Worry.** Children have vivid imaginations, especially when they are fueled by disrupted households and whispered conversations between parents. Age-appropriate, verbal explanations can help children be more realistic about what happens at the hospital,

*I am the first of four children and the only girl. When I was diagnosed with leukemia at the age of fourteen, it affected all our lives. My brother Wes was thirteen, Matthew was four and Erik was two. They and my parents were my support system.*

*Wes was my support at home and school. He stuck up for me and kept an eye on me. Matt and Erik would accompany my mom and me to treatments and hold my hand. If one of them wasn't with me when I went in, the nurses would ask where they were. These little boys made it easier for me to be brave.*

but nothing is as powerful as a visit. The effectiveness of a visit will depend on your child's age and temperament, but many parents say bringing the siblings along helps everyone. The sibling gains an accurate understanding of hospital procedures, the sick child is comforted by the presence of the sibling, and parents get to spend time with all their children.

Allowing even the youngest children to help the family can reduce siblings' worries. When children have clear explanations of the situation, and concrete jobs to do that benefit the family, they tend to rise to the occasion.

• **Concern about parents.** Parents focused on helping their sick child get through an illness or injury often are not aware of their healthy children's strong feelings. They sometimes assume that children understand that they are loved, and would get the same attention if they were sick or injured. But siblings often do not share their feelings of anger, jealousy, or worry because they do not want to place additional burdens on their parents. It is all too common to hear siblings say, "I have to be the strong one. I don't want to cause my parents any more pain." But burdens are lighter if shared, and parents should try to encourage all their children to talk about how they are feeling.

# Helping siblings cope

Being available to listen, to say, "I hear how painful this is for you," or, "You sound scared. I am, too," makes siblings feel they are still valued members of the family and, even though their sick or injured brother or sister is absorbing the lion's share of parents' time and care, they are still cherished.

You can help siblings of a sick or injured child by keeping them involved, making sure they know they

*I'm fifteen now. Looking back at my brother's long illness, the parts I hated the most were: not understanding what was being done to him, answering endless worried phone calls, and hearing the answers to my own questions when my parents talked to other people.*

are loved, and addressing any problems that develop.

- Make sure that all the children clearly understand the nature of the illness or injury. If an illness is contagious, ask your doctor about special precautions and explain these to the whole family.

- Seek ways to keep mothers and toddlers together—such separations are very difficult. When mothers must leave to go to the hospital, they sometimes leave out family photo albums for the caregiver to show the toddler whenever she gets sad.

- Have scheduled family meetings to help the family function during the crisis. These times can be used to update everyone on the medical situation, air complaints, and make plans for fun.

> Kim's hospitalizations were very hard on five-year-old Kelly. My parents kept Kelly during the week, so this helped a lot. Dennis would pick her up after work. I remember being at the hospital all week long, then Dennis would come on the weekends and I would go home and do things with Kelly. We would go out to eat, or go roller-skating. I really missed her and it was just so hard on everyone. I remember being so tired, but I feel that you need to spend time with all of your children because they need you also.

- Try to spend time individually with each sibling: take a trip, see a movie, or ride bicycles together.

- Bring up siblings when people focus only on the sick child. For example, if someone exclaims, "Oh look how good Lisa looks," you could say, "Yes, and Martha has a new haircut, too. Don't you like it?"

- Include siblings in decision-making. Let them choose how to parcel out extra chores. Or devise a schedule for parent time with the healthy children.

- Alert siblings' teachers about the stress at home. Many children respond to worries about illness or injury by developing behavior or academic problems at school. Ask teachers to watch for warning signals, and provide extra support or tutoring. Communicate frequently with siblings' teachers and try to stay abreast of any developing problems.

- Expect siblings to develop some behavior problems if your child's illness or injury is long-term. This is normal.

- Give siblings gifts and tokens of appreciation for helping out during hard times. Encourage your sick child to share the many toys and gifts he receives to prevent hurt feelings or jealousy.

- Encourage a close relationship between an adult relative or neighbor and your other children. Having someone special around when parents are absent can prevent problems and help your child feel cared for and loved.

- Give lots of hugs and kisses.

## Positive outcomes

Many siblings don't have problems when a brother or sister is sick or injured. Often they exhibit great warmth and active caretaking while their sibling is in the hospital, and develop true empathy and compassion. Afterward, some brothers and sisters say they have increased knowledge about disease, increased empathy for the sick or disabled, an increased sense of responsibility, enhanced self-esteem, greater maturity and coping ability, and increased family closeness. Many of these siblings mature into adults interested in the caring professions such as medicine, social work, or teaching.

*I think it is important for parents to think about the needs of the siblings and discuss creative ways to meet those needs. However, we must also remember that children are self-centered little beings who need and desire attention. Sibling rivalry will always be present. Parents need to consider everyone's needs, and then do the best they can. I think parents should feel proud, rather than guilty, that under the most difficult of circumstances, they portioned themselves out as fairly as possible.*

# CHAPTER FOURTEEN

# Long-Term Illness: Keeping Family Life Going

*Life can only be understood backwards;*
*however it must be lived forwards.*

—*Soren Kierkegaard*

AFTER A SHORT-TERM ILLNESS OR INJURY, most families return to normal routines quickly. But caring for a sick or hurt child can severely disrupt family life when treatment or recovery takes more than a few weeks. This chapter contains some suggestions for dealing with lifestyle and behavior changes that may accompany long-term illness or injury.

## Taking care of yourself

You can run yourselves ragged when your child is in the hospital. Try to find one or two ways to stay healthy and balanced.

- Strive to eat, sleep, and get a few minutes of exercise every day.

- Take turns staying with your child at night. If the hospital is far from home, you could rent a hotel room nearby, stay in a Ronald McDonald House or hospital hospitality house, or borrow a mobile home or trailer to park at the hospital. A refuge from the noise and smells of a hospital can be a welcome, and needed, relief.

> *Whenever Brent was in the hospital, we both wanted to be there. During his second extended stay in the hospital, we both let go a little, and we each took turns sleeping at the Ronald McDonald House. That way we each got a decent night's sleep (or some sleep) every other night.*

- Ask a favorite aunt, uncle, or grandparent to spend nights at the hospital occasionally so both parents can go home to sleep. This can be especially comforting for siblings.

- Find ways to vent your feelings about the hospitalization. You can talk with a spouse, another parent at the hospital, a friend, a family member, or a counselor.

# Work

When both parents work, they must decide what to do about their jobs. If you can, use all available sick leave and vacation days before you decide whether one parent should leave a job. You also need to evaluate your financial situation and insurance availability. This requires time and clarity of thought; both are in short supply when your child is ill.

In August 1993, the Family and Medical Leave Act (FMLA) became federal law. The act protects job security of workers in large companies (50+ employees within a 75 mile radius) who must take a leave of absence for many medical reasons, including caring for a seriously ill child, recovering from a medical condition, giving birth, or adopting a child. Consult your employee handbook or personnel director about your organization's policies.

Federal law also protects your insurance for eighteen months after you leave your job, but you will have to pay the premiums.

> *My husband and I shared decision-making by keeping a joint medical journal. The days that my husband stayed at the hospital, he would write down all medicines given, side effects, fever, vital signs, food consumed, sleep patterns, and any questions that needed to be asked at the next rounds. This way, I knew exactly what had been happening. Decisions were made as we traded shifts at our son's bedside.*

# Marriage

Long-term medical treatments and conditions that are life-threatening to a child can place enormous pressures on a marriage. Couples can be separated for long periods of time, emotions are high, and coping styles and skills differ. Couples must survive this difficult period, then work together to rearrange their lives in a new pattern. Working together to handle the situation can help immensely.

- Share medical decisions.

- Take turns staying in the hospital with your ill child.

- Share responsibility for home care.

- Make spending time together a priority, even if it is only thirty minutes a day for coffee in the hospital cafeteria.

- Accept differences in coping styles.

- Seek counseling.

*My husband and I went to counseling to try to work out a way to split up the child rearing and household duties because I was overwhelmed and resenting it. I guess it helped a little bit, but the best thing that came out of it was that I kept seeing the counselor by myself. My son wanted to go to the "feelings doctor," too. I received a lot of very helpful, practical advice on the many behavior problems my son developed. And my son had an objective, safe person to talk things over with.*

Marriages with existing troubles usually are most strained by caring for a gravely ill child. If serious conflicts develop, don't hesitate to seek outside help. Most marriages survive a child's serious illness or injury, but some don't.

# Divorced parents

Parents who were separated or divorced prior to their child's injury or illness face additional difficulties. They will have to work together to help their child.

- Agree to set aside differences for the duration of the crisis.

- Focus on communication.

- Make agreements and abide by them.

- Go to mediation if conflicts cannot be resolved.

Anything divorced parents can do to prevent or minimize stress will help their child physically and emotionally.

# Parents' reactions

Some parents have no major problems coping with a sick or hurt child. They find unexpected reserves of strength and ask for help from their friends and family when they need it. They realize that family members' needs change during stressful times and they alter

> *I lost thirty-five pounds in the first six weeks of my son's hospitalization. I had almost constant diarrhea and vomited frequently.*

their expectations and parenting accordingly. These families usually had strong and effective communication prior to the illness, and pull together as a unit to deal with it. But most parents experience a range of emotional and physical reactions to their child's serious illness.

- **Illness.** Parents watching over children in the hospital often fail to eat and sleep. They become so focused on their child's health that they neglect their own. So it's not surprising that parents of children in the hospital often become ill themselves.

- **Confusion and numbness.** When a child is injured or very ill, parents often experience shock, followed by confusion and numbness. This is a normal reaction: the mind tries to block out painful information. The confusion will pass, but parents may need to take extra time to jot down information that they normal-

> *I felt so bad that Aurora was in such obvious pain and there was really nothing I could do. As a parent, there's a part of you that would take that pain into your own body.*

ly wouldn't have trouble remembering.

- **Denial**. Parents faced with a seriously ill or injured child may experience denial. This, too, is a common response.

- **Guilt**. Parents often blame themselves for their child's illness or injury. They wonder what they could have done to prevent the situation: How could I have kept her from climbing that tree? Should I have let him drink the well water?

- **Fear and hopelessness**. A hospital has a routine of its own: every staff member has defined tasks and clear duties, while parents may feel helpless. Many parents say they feel more powerful when they establish a new routine and begin helping their child cope.

- **Anger**. Anger is a typical response to a child's illness or injury. Sometimes parents vent their anger on hospital staff or their family and friends. To cope with anger, parents should learn healthy ways to vent, including discussing feelings, exercising, crying in the shower, pounding the walls, or seeking counseling.

- **Sadness and grief**. Even when the child is expected to recover fully, parents may experience sadness and grief about their child's trauma. This is normal.

- **Hope**. Hope is the belief in a better tomorrow. Hope sustains the will to live and gives the strength to endure each trial. Cultivating

> *I'm a controlled person. My four-year-old needed me to show I was upset, too. One day, after a blood draw, she yelled at me all the way to the car saying, "You just want them to hurt me; you don't love me; why do you take me to get hurt?" I sat in the car and burst into tears. I told her bringing her for pokes was the hardest thing I'd ever done. That I wished it was me instead. That I loved her so much and wanted to protect her from hurt, but I couldn't. I told her that I wanted her to get better and we just had to get through the treatment. She looked at me, patted me on the arm, and said, "It's okay now Mom, let's just go home."*

a hopeful attitude will help you cope with your child's extended hospitalization—one day at a time.

# Behavior changes under extreme stress

When a child is sick or hurt, parents experience physical, emotional, financial, and spiritual stress. A crisis can bring many negative behaviors to the surface.

- **Dishonesty.** As stated earlier, children feel safe when their parents are honest with them. If parents keep secrets from children, or try to protect them from bad news, they feel isolated and fearful. A child might think, "If Mom and Dad won't tell me, it must be really bad," or, "Mom won't talk about it. I guess there's nobody that I can tell about how scared I am."

- **Denial.** Denial is a type of unconscious dishonesty. This occurs when parents say, "Everything will be just fine," or, "It won't hurt a bit." This type of pretending increases the distance between child and parent, leaving the child with no support. However horrible the truth, it seldom is as terrifying as a half-truth upon which a child's imagination builds.

- **Depression.** Depression is common among parents of seriously hurt or sick children. Parents should seek professional help if they regularly experience any of the following symptoms: changes in sleeping patterns (sleeping too much, waking up frequently during the night, early morning awakening), appetite disturbances (eating too little or too much), loss of sex drive, fatigue, panic attacks, inability to experience pleasure, feelings of sadness and despair, poor concentration, social withdrawal, feelings of worth-

*When my daughter became very sick, I bought her everything that I saw that was pretty and lovely. I kept thinking that, if she died, she would die happy because she'd be surrounded by all these beautiful things. Even when I couldn't really afford it, I kept buying. I realize now that I was doing it to make me feel better, not her. She needed cuddling and loving, not clothes and dolls.*

lessness, suicidal thoughts, drug or alcohol abuse. Depressed parents often neglect their children's needs. Depression is common and treatable. A therapist can treat depression with counseling, medication, or both.

- **Showing no emotion or too much emotion.** Either extreme can frighten children. Children can become angry at parents who show too little emotion because they fear their parents don't care about their pain. But children also can withdraw from parents who show too much emotion. They need parents who admit that they hurt, too, but are willing to face the fears and pain with their child.

*I realized that I had formed a habit of treating my child as if she were still young and sick. One day, when I was pouring her juice, I thought, "Why am I doing this? She's seven. She needs to learn to make her own sandwiches and pour her own drinks. She needs to be encouraged to grow up." Boy, it has been hard. But I've stuck to my guns, and made other extended family members do it, too. I want her to grow up to be an independent adult, not a demanding, overgrown kid.*

- **Loss of temper.** All parents lose their tempers sometimes. They lose their tempers with spouses, healthy children, pets, even strangers. But anger can be especially painful when the target is a sick child. If stressed, parents can give themselves a ten-minute quiet time in private to regroup. If, despite their best efforts, parents find they are too stressed to control their tempers, a professional counselor can help them explore new ways of coping.

- **Unequal application of household rules.** Parents guarantee family problems if the ill child enjoys favored status while the siblings must do extra chores. It is hard to know when to insist that an ill child resume making his bed or setting the table, but it must be done. Siblings should know from the very beginning that any child in the family, if sick, will be excused from chores, but must start again when he is able.

- **Overindulgence.** Parents often overindulge sick or injured children, and sometimes are reluctant to teach the child life skills.

- **Overprotection.** Parents should ask the doctor what changes in physical activity are necessary for safety and not impose restrictions that go beyond this. Letting children become involved in sports or neighborhood play may be difficult, but it helps them feel better as well as develop friendships.

# CHAPTER FIFTEEN

# School

*Education is an ornament in prosperity
and a refuge in adversity.*

—*Aristotle*

SICK OR INJURED CHILDREN OFTEN EXPERIENCE disruptions in their education. These can range from a few missed lessons to long-term absences caused by repeated hospitalizations or side effects from medication.

Returning to school can be either a relief or a major challenge if your child has missed weeks or months of school. For many children, going back to school signals a return to normal life. Other children, especially teens, may dread returning to school because of changes in appearance, learning ability, or concerns that prolonged absences may have changed their social standing with their friends.

Most of the information in this chapter deals with schooling for children with a long-term illness or repeated hospitalizations. Educating these children can become complicated, but usually can be successfully managed through planning and good communication.

## Keep the school informed

If your child will miss more than a week or two of school, you should find someone to act as liaison with hospital, family, and school. The advocate will keep information flowing between the hospital and school, and will help pave the way for your child's successful return to class. The hospital social worker often acts as the advocate, but a school nurse, psychologist, principal, or other motivated individual also can step into this role. The most important qualifications for this role are good communication skills, knowledge of educational programs and procedures, comfort in dealing with school issues, and organizational skills. Choose someone you trust to act fairly on your child's behalf.

The advocate should locate a contact person at the school (or hospital) and provide frequent updates about your child's medical condition, treatment, emotional state, and tentative reentry date. The advocate should encourage questions, and address staff concerns about having a sick child in school.

> *We had absolutely no problem keeping the school informed as we lived directly behind it. The teacher would frequently stop by on her way home to drop off homework assignments and cards or messages from Stephan's classmates. The school nurse, psychologist, and teacher were at my beck and call. Whenever I felt that we needed to talk, I'd call and they would set up a meeting within twenty-four hours. They have been wonderful.*

## Keep teachers and classmates involved

Your child's well-being in the hospital depends, in part, on staying connected with his teacher and classmates. The teacher should receive regular updates through the advocate, but you can help by calling the teacher periodically, and bringing notes or taped messages to the classroom. If your child is in middle or high school, all of her teachers should receive this information.

- Seek out brief, easy-to-digest information about your child's illness. Give the materials to the teacher for information or to share with the class.

- Have the nurse or social worker come to class to give a presentation about what is happening to their classmate and how he will look and feel when he returns. This should include a question and answer session to clear up misconceptions and allay fears.

Teenagers should be involved in any decisions about information to be given to classmates.

- Encourage classmates to keep in touch by sending notes, calling on the telephone, sending class pictures, or making a banner. (Other ideas are contained in the chapter, *Families and Friends: How to Help.*)

# Keep up with schoolwork

Keeping up with schoolwork usually can help your child stay connected to her everyday routine. You can communicate with the teacher to keep abreast of subjects being covered in school. Often, the teacher will send assignments and materials home with siblings, or you can make arrangements for someone to pick them up. Friends or relatives can volunteer to be tutors. They can provide a much-needed link to the school and give you a welcome break.

*We have worked to educate ourselves and our son about his heart problems. Now, if David gets teased at the beginning of the school year, he tells the class exactly what's wrong with his heart. He's very open and truthful about it and they respect him for it. They are nicer after he tells them. They can respect his differences and understand why he is the way he is.*

Some states require school districts to provide hospital tutoring when children are hospitalized for long stays. Most large children's hospitals have teachers on staff, as well as educational liaisons who can help you work out appropriate schooling.

Parents should consider alternative learning activities if children are struggling with schoolwork because of fatigue or illness. Parents and children can identify areas of special interest, such as space travel or animals. Children often learn reading, math, and other skills more readily if they are in the context of a topic they find interesting. Parents should discuss such approaches with teachers who often can provide valuable resources and support.

# Returning to school

The sooner a child can return to school, the better. Preparation and communication are key to a successful return. If your child has only missed a week or two, work with the teacher to find ways for your child to catch up. If, however, your child has been gone for an extended period, ask the physician or primary nurse to prepare a letter for the school staff containing the following information:

> My high-school gym teacher gave me a B after I tore the ligament in my knee and had surgery. Even though I was able to lift weights during class, I couldn't participate in regular class activities. In hindsight, I should have fought this or negotiated to drop the class and take it again later.

- The student's health status and its probable effect on attendance.

- Whether he can attend regular physical education classes, physical education with restrictions (no running, for example), or adaptive physical education.

- Whether adjustments in your child's schedule are needed. For example, a child with a cast on his arm will be unable to complete a typing class and may benefit from changing classes, even if this isn't standard school procedure.

- A description of any changes in physical appearance, perhaps with suggestions on how to discuss this with classmates.

- The possible effect of medications on academic performance.

- Whether school personnel must administer medications or other services as directed by a doctor.

- A reminder to never give any medication, even aspirin, without parental permission.

- Any special considerations such as extra snacks, rest periods, or extra time to get from class to class.

- Whether exposure to communicable disease could harm your child.

- A list of signs and symptoms requiring parent notification, such as fever, nausea, pain, swelling, or nosebleeds.

Stress that the teacher's job is to teach, and the parent and school nurse will take care of all medical issues.

Once teachers have had a chance to read the letter, request a meeting that includes faculty, administrators, school nurse, and school counselor or psychologist. At this meeting, answer any questions about the information contained in the letter, pass out any useful information you have, and do your best to establish a rapport with the entire staff. Take this opportunity to express appreciation for the school's help and your hopes for a close collaboration in the future to create a supportive climate for your child.

The following are additional parent suggestions on how to prevent problems through preparation and communication:

> *I'm a school nurse. I like parents and their children to come and talk with me when it's time for the child to reenter school. We talk about: how the child is feeling, how many hours a day he should be in school, whether he needs to come rest in my office. I remind parents that I need doctor's orders to give meds or provide nursing services. I love it when parents share information through conversation, journal articles, or brochures. I also prepare the child's class for reentry. I give talks and show videos. I find children to be wonderfully receptive and helpful when they are given truthful information.*

- Keep the school informed and involved from the beginning. This fosters a spirit that "we're all in this together."

- Reassure the staff that, even if the child looks frail, he really belongs in school.

- If your child has a long-term illness, bring the nurse into the class whenever necessary to talk about your child's illness or injury and answer questions.

- Ask the school to bend some rules and policies if you think it will help your youngster.

- Find ways to check your child's progress when she returns. Some children, especially teens, are reluctant to talk about school with parents, but they may need a parent's help negotiating changes in school schedules or rules.

> *When Brent returned to kindergarten after a long stay in the hospital, he was often exhausted. There was a beanbag chair in the back of his classroom, and he just curled up in it and went to sleep when he needed to.*

- Consider renting or buying a cellular telephone so that the school can contact you if any problems arise, there are any questions, or your child needs to leave school due to fatigue or illness.

- Volunteer at school if you feel it is important to be nearby in case of problems.

- Realize that teachers and other school staff can be frightened, overwhelmed, and discouraged when they have a child with a serious illness in their classroom. Accurate information and words of appreciation can help immensely.

# Siblings and school

Siblings can be overlooked while parents deal with a sick or hurt child. Many siblings keep their feelings bottled up inside to prevent placing additional burdens on their parents. Often, their stress is most obvious at school.

Some parents occasionally allow their healthy siblings to play hooky to be with the ill child in the hospital or to stay at home to rest. The emotional connection between brothers and sisters is important to their well-being.

Remember to include the siblings' teachers in all conferences at school. They should be told about the stresses facing the family and

*Lindsey was in kinder-
garten when Jesse first got
sick. Because we heard
nothing from the kinder-
garten teacher, we
assumed that things were
going well. At the end of
the year, the teacher told
us that Lindsey frequently
spent part of each day hid-
ing under her desk. When
I asked why we had never
been told, the teacher said
she thought that we
already had enough to
worry about dealing with
Jesse's illness and treatment. She was wrong to
make decisions for us, but
I wish we had been more
attentive. Lindsey needed
help.*

understand that feelings may bubble to the surface in their classroom.

If your child has an emergency or medical setback, notify your healthy children's teachers so they can give extra attention and be alert for signs of stress. Encourage school personnel to ask the siblings, "I know your brother is very sick, but how are you doing?"

# CHAPTER SIXTEEN

# Keeping Medical Records

*Life is a grindstone. But whether it grinds us down
or polishes us up depends on us.*

—L. Thomas Holdcroft

KEEPING TRACK OF MEDICAL PAPERWORK is a necessary evil. Think of yourself as someone with two sets of books, the hospital's and your own. If the hospital loses your child's chart or misplaces lab results, you will still have your own records. If your child's chart becomes a foot thick, you will have a system that makes it easy to spot trends and retrieve dosage information.

Parents should record:

- Dates and results of all lab work.
- Dates of treatments, including drugs given, and dose.
- All changes in dosages of medicine.
- All side effects from drugs.
- Any fevers or illnesses.
- Dates of all medical appointments and the names of the doctors seen.
- Dates of any procedures done.
- Child's sleeping patterns, appetite, and emotions.

If your child has an emergency illness or injury, you may not be able to keep

*For a long time I was unorganized, which is very unlike the way I usually am. I found that my usual excellent memory just wasn't working well.
It all seemed to run together, and I began to forget if I had given her all of her pills. Then I began using a calendar for medications. I wrote every med on the correct days, then checked them off as I gave them.*

records as described. Try to at least record what procedures and surgeries occurred, and the names of the doctors providing the service. This allows you to check your bills for accuracy later.

There are as many good ways to record medical information as there are parents.

- Journal. Keeping a notebook works extremely well for people who like to write. Parents make entries every day about all pertinent medical information and often include personal information, such as their feelings or memorable things their child says. Journals are easy to carry back and forth to the clinic, and can be written in while waiting for appointments. They also have the advantage of having unlimited space. One disadvantage is that they can be misplaced.

> *I had a paper and pen sitting right there by Chase and every now and again I picked it up and wrote something. Some days it was just my thoughts and feelings. Other days I wrote down details of Chase's treatment. Some days I wrote down things like, "Chase is really cranky today," or, "He's running a high temperature." I actually had doctors write in my journal if I couldn't spell something or I wanted them to explain the treatment. It really helped.*

- Calendar. For simple illnesses, you can probably use a calendar you already have for appointments. For lengthy or complex illnesses, you can buy a new calendar just for recording medical information and hang it next to the telephone or in another convenient place. You can record test results and other data on the calendar while talking to the nurse or lab technician on the phone, and take it with you to all appointments.

- Hospital-supplied charts. Many hospitals supply folders containing photocopied sheets for record-keeping.

- Three ring binder and hole punch. A good method to keep copies of lab reports, discharge orders, consent forms, hospital admission forms, and other hospital paperwork.

- **Tape recorder.** A tape recorder works well if you keep track of more information than a calendar can hold, or find writing a journal too time-consuming. Small machines are very inexpensive, and can be carried in a pocket.

- **Computer.** For the computer-literate, keeping all medical and financial records on the computer is an attractive option. You can take a laptop or electronic datebook to the hospital and enter hospital information there.

Your records will help pull information together and keep it straight. They will help you remember questions, prevent mistakes, notice trends. They will help busy doctors remember what happened the last time your child was given a certain drug. Your records will help the entire medical team give your child the best possible care.

# CHAPTER SEVENTEEN

# Hospital Billing

*Nothing in the world can take the place of persistence.*
—*Calvin Coolidge*

BILLS CAN BE ONE OF THE LASTING NIGHTMARES of hospital stays. Even when you have good insurance and your child's hospital stay is short, it pays to keep good records, stay alert for billing inaccuracies, and get problems resolved quickly. Even bills for short stays or simple procedures can quickly reach very large amounts.

When treatment is long and complex, the potential for errors escalates and the consequences of not having records or of ignoring problems can be financially devastating. For all families, knowing what expenses are tax-deductible will help you keep the necessary records now and potentially save money at tax time.

## Keeping financial records

Accurate records are a necessary defense against hospital overbilling. Poor organization of bills can mean you will be hounded by collection companies. However, many simple systems exist for keeping financial records.

For most financial records, you will need just an expandable folder. If your child's illness involves many or

> I go through every bill looking for errors. At one point David had angioplasty and catheterization. The hospital part of the bill came to twenty thousand dollars. By the time I was done with the bill, it was only nine thousand dollars because I found so many errors.

lengthy hospitalizations, you will probably need a well-organized file cabinet. Financial records are a major headache for many parents, but keeping organized records can prevent financial problems that affect your credit or keep you from being able to support your family's other wants and needs.

- Whenever you open an envelope containing medical billing or insurance information, file the contents immediately. Don't put it on a pile or throw it in a drawer.

- Keep a notebook with a running log of all tax-deductible medical expenses, including the service, charge, bill paid, date paid, and check number.

- Don't pay a bill unless you have checked over each item listed to make sure that it is correct.

- Set up a file cabinet just for medical expense records. Have hanging files for hospital bills, doctor bills, all other medical bills, insurance explanations of benefits (EOB), prescription receipts, tax deductible receipts (tolls, parking, motels, meals), and correspondence.

> *The hospital where my daughter received her radiation gave me a folder the first day. It included a sheet giving all the information for preventing and solving billing problems. I never needed to call because the hospital billing was clear, prompt, and organized.*
>
> *The hospital where she was a frequent inpatient and clinic patient billed from three different departments, put charges from the same visit on different bills, overbilled, made errors, and threatened to send the account to collections. It was a never-ending grind and a constant frustration.*

# Hospital billing problems

Not everyone experiences billing problems. People who have managed health care plans or receive public assistance may never see bills. Other parents have no problems with billing throughout their child's treatment. But many parents of children who spend time in the hospital encounter billing problems.

- Keep all records filed in an organized fashion.

- Check every bill from the hospital to make sure there are no charges for treatments not given or errors, such as double billing.

- Check to see if the hospital has financial counselors. If so, make contact early in your child's hospitalization. Counselors provide services in many areas, including help with understanding the hospital's billing system, billing insurance carriers, understanding explanations of benefits, hospital and insurance correspondence, dealing with Medicaid, working out a payment plan, designing a ledger system for tracking insurance claims, and resolving disputes.

*After about twenty phone calls to the director of billing, I finally said to her secretary, "You know, I have a desperately sick child here, and I have more important things to do than call your boss every day. I've been as patient and polite as I can. What else can I do?" She said, "Honey, get irate. It works every time." I told her to put me through to somebody, anybody, and I would. She connected me to the person who mediates disputes, I got irate, and we went through all the bills line by line.*

- Compare each hospital bill to the explanation of benefits (EOB) you receive from your insurance company. Track down discrepancies.

- Call the hospital immediately if you find a billing error. Write down the date, the name of the person you talk to, and the plan of action.

- Call and talk to the billing supervisor if the error is not corrected on your next bill. Explain politely the steps you have already taken and how you would like the problem fixed.

- Write a brief letter to the billing supervisor if the problem is not corrected. Explain the steps you have taken and request immediate action. Keep a copy of each letter you write.

- Ask the hospital billing department and your insurance company, in writing, to audit your account if you are inundated with a constant stream of bills and there are major discrepancies between the hospital charges and your records of treatment given. This is a common practice. Insist on a line-by-line explanation for each charge.

- Ask a family member or friend to help if you are too tired or overwhelmed to deal with the bills. He could come every other week, open and file all bills and insurance papers, make phone calls, and write all necessary letters. Friends also can enter your records in a computer.

- Don't let billing problems accumulate. Your account may end up at a collection agency, which can quickly become a huge headache.

*Within five months of my daughter's diagnosis, the billing was so messed up that I despaired of ever getting it straight. When the hospital threatened to send the account to a collection agency, I took action. I wrote letters to the hospital and the insurance company demanding an audit. When both audits arrived, they were thousands of dollars apart. I met with our insurance representative. She called the hospital, and we had a three-way showdown. We straightened it out that time, but every bill that I received for the duration of treatment had one or more errors, always in the hospital's favor.*

## Deductible medical expenses

Insurance may not cover many expenses, including gas, car repairs, motels, food away from home, health insurance deducibles, and prescriptions. Many of these items can be deducted from your federal income tax. To find out what can be legally deducted while your child undergoes medical treatment, get IRS publication 502. This booklet is available at many libraries and most IRS offices or by calling 1-800-TAX-FORM (1-800-829-3676) from 8 A.M. to 5 P.M. weekdays and 9 A.M. to 3 P.M. Saturdays.

Families of children with life-threatening conditions, such as premature births, can easily spend much of their income on items not covered by insurance. Often parents are too exhausted to go through stacks of bills at the end of the year to calculate deductions. Keep a running list of bills, and write down the total in a notebook each month. Then, all you need to do at tax time is add up the monthly totals.

You can easily keep track of tax-deductible items by gluing an envelope to the inside cover of your calendar. Whenever you incur a tax-deductible expense, put the receipt in the envelope, and file it when you get home.

# CHAPTER EIGHTEEN

# Insurance

*Be it better or be it worse*
*Please you the man that bears the purse.*

—Thomas Delaney

FINDING ONE'S WAY THROUGH THE INSURANCE MAZE can be a difficult task. Understanding the benefits and claims procedures, however, will help you get the bills paid without undue stress.

## Understand your policy

Read your entire insurance manual to learn the details of your coverage. Make a list of any questions you have about terms or benefits. With a managed care plan, you may have a limited network of providers, and hefty penalties or no benefits if you go outside the network. Your policy should tell you:

- Your deductible, the amount of money you must pay before insurance coverage begins.

- Whether your coverage increases to 100 percent when costs reach a certain point.

- Whether there is a lifetime limit on benefits.

- When a second opinion is required.

*I realized that my daughter had been treated for over four months and I had never called the insurance company. When I read the manual, I was horrified to find out that I had not prenotified them about three hospitalizations. There was a two hundred dollar penalty for each lapse. I called in tears, and they only charged me for one mistake, not all three.*

- When you have to notify the company about hospitalizations. Many firms require notification before treatment, except in the case of emergency.

- Whether you qualify for home nursing care. If so, check to see how many visits are covered.

If you expect many hospitalizations, get a copy of every form you might need, such as claim forms for inpatient care, outpatient care, or prescriptions. You can cut down on paperwork by filling in all the subscriber information on one of each type of form (except date and signature) and then making many copies. You will have a form ready to send in with each bill.

# Find a contact person

If your child has a long-term illness or an injury that requires many treatments, call your insurance company and ask who will handle your claims. Explain the situation to your insurance representatives and tell them it would be helpful to always deal with the same person. Insurers sometimes can assign you a contact person to review claims, handle special needs, and answer any questions that you have about benefits. Try to develop a cooperative relationship with your contact person because she can make your life much easier. Your employer may also have a benefits person who can operate as a liaison with the insurer.

Don't be afraid to negotiate benefits with the insurance company. Your contact person sometimes can redefine a service that your child needs so it will be covered.

*Our insurance company covered 100 percent of maintenance drugs only if the patient needed them for the rest of their lives. Christine's drugs were only needed for two years but were extremely expensive. I asked my contact person for help, and she petitioned the decision-making board. They granted us an exemption and covered the entire cost of all her maintenance drugs.*

# Challenging a claim

You can obtain maximum benefit from your insurance policy by keeping accurate records and challenging any claims your provider denies.

- Make photocopies of everything you send to your insurance company, including claims, letters, and bills.

- Pay bills by check, and keep all canceled checks.

- Keep all correspondence you receive from billing and insurance companies.

- Write down the date, the name of the person contacted, and details of all telephone conversations related to insurance.

- Keep accurate records of all medical expenses and claims you submit.

Policyholders have a right to appeal claims their insurance company denies.

- Keep original documents in your files, and send photocopies to the insurance company with a letter outlining why you think the claim should be covered. Demand a written reply.

- Talk to your state's insurance commissioner (or other office with similar duties) to learn how to file a complaint. Find out what power the state has to help you resolve your dispute.

*My daughter went to the hospital clinic every three months for an examination and IV medication. Over the two year period, each bill was different, ranging from $329 to $740, for identical treatments! I told the insurance company not to pay any bills until I had confirmed their accuracy. I called the billing supervisor so often that we were on a first name basis. I always tried to be upbeat and we laughed a lot. She stopped investigating every problem and would just delete the charge from the computer. But I resented the time and energy it took to constantly correct the mistakes.*

- Contact your congressional delegation. All senators and members of the House of Representatives have staff members who help constituents with problems.

- Take your claim to small claims court or hire an attorney skilled in insurance matters to sue the insurance company if you've exhausted all other means to resolve the dispute.

Don't be afraid to ask questions and be persistent.

# CHAPTER NINETEEN

# Sources of Financial Help

*Lack of money is trouble without equal.*

*—Rabelais*

SOURCES OF FINANCIAL ASSISTANCE VARY from state to state and town to town. To track down possible sources, ask the hospital social worker for help. Some hospitals also have community outreach nurses or case workers who may point out potential sources of assistance.

## Hospital policy

If you are unable to pay your hospital bills, do not let your account go to a collection agency or take out a large loan to pay the bill. Ask the hospital social worker to set up an appointment for you with the appropriate person to discuss your hospital's financial assistance policy. Many hospitals write off a percentage of the cost of care if the patient is uninsured or underinsured.

## Supplemental Security Income

Supplemental Security Income (SSI) is a source of financial help based on family income. The Social Security Administration administers the program. Recipients must be ill, blind, or disabled, with a low family income. Children with some types of illness or injury may qualify as disabled for this program, making them eligible for monthly aid if the family income is low enough.

To find out if your child qualifies, look in the telephone book under "United States Government" for the "Social Security Administration." Ask to speak to someone regarding eligibility for SSI. If eligible, you may need to travel to the nearest office to apply.

If this is a hardship, the caseworker will take your application over the telephone.

# Medicaid

State governments administer Medicaid and the federal government pays a portion. Eligibility rules vary from state to state, but families with private insurance sometimes are eligible if huge hospital bills are only partially covered. Your local or county social service department can give you the number for the Medicaid office in your area.

In addition to helping pay some or all hospital bills, Medicaid sometimes also pays transportation and prescription costs. Some states cover children under the age of twenty-one if they are hospitalized for more than thirty days, regardless of parental income. Ask for a detailed list of benefits available in your state.

# Free medicine programs

Many drug companies have programs that provide free medicines to needy patients. Eligibility requirements vary, but most are available to those not covered by private or public insurance programs. Ask your physician to request, on letterhead, a free copy of the Pharmaceutical Industry Patient Assistance Directory from:

Pharmaceutical Manufacturers Association
1100 15th Street NW
Washington, DC 20005
Toll-free hot line for physicians: 1-800-PMA-INFO

# Service organizations

Many service organizations help families in need. They can provide transportation, special equipment, or food. Often, all a family has to do is describe their plight, and good Samaritans appear. Some organizations that may have chapters in your community are: American Legion; Elks Club; fraternal organizations such as Masons, Jaycees, Kiwanis Club, Knights of Columbus, Lions,

Rotary; United Way; Veterans of Foreign Wars; and churches of all denominations. Local philanthropic organizations also help needy families in many communities. To find them, call your local health department, speak to the social worker, and ask for help.

# Fund raising and special help

Many communities rally around a sick child by organizing a fund. Help can range from collection jars in local stores to an organized drive using the local media. Fundraising has many pitfalls and you should take great care to protect the privacy of the sick child. If you are contemplating starting a fund, read Sheila Peterson's *A Special Way to Care*, listed in the *Resources* section of this book. This guide gives detailed, step-by-step advice on determining the needs of the family, finding benefits, using publicity, generating community support, and managing the fund.

CHAPTER TWENTY

# Looking Back

*Time cools, time clarifies.*

—*Thomas Mann*

HOSPITAL STAYS CAN BE physically and emotionally challenging for children, siblings, parents, family, and friends. But, from facing and dealing with adversity comes change and, often, growth. The dozens of parents who shared their stories in this book described many benefits and positive aftereffects for all members of the family.

Children who have short stays or outpatient procedures, report learning:

- The type of work that doctors and nurses do.
- How their body works.
- The types of medical problems that other children face.
- How to handle a difficult or painful experience.

The lives of families of children who endure long or frequent hospitalizations are often changed forever. These parents, children, and siblings describe many long-lasting benefits from their experiences.

- **Appreciation.** Looking back, many parents reflected on the people they met. They describe kids with incredible courage, parents they will never forget, and caregivers who just never stopped giving. The people they met in hospitals whose situations were very grave bestowed a renewed appreciation for life. They now cherish the little things: their child's smile, the first hug of the day, the morning sun. Life slows down, and is savored.

- **Awareness.** Parents described the incredible intensity of their child's hospital experience. One mother said, "So much happened so quickly, and was so emotionally powerful, that we felt like we were in a true life drama unfolding in the hospital room." The emotions experienced by children and parents alike changed their awareness of normal. Life seemed fuller and richer than in the past.

- **Bonding.** Sharing a hospital experience, day and night, with your child can forge close bonds. It gives parents and child time together, to talk, to play, sometimes to laugh. Children realize the enormity of their parent's love, and parents often become closer to their children simply by sharing a room and focusing all of their attention on their child.

- **Emotions.** Parents shared that the experience of living through a serious illness and hospitalization brought their emotions closer to the surface. They cry more and they laugh louder. They learned to make every day count and to weave wonderful memories out of little things the family shared. Hugs became valuable, and, many years later, they still hug each other more. They learned to reach out and show people how much they care.

- **Knowledge of the medical system.** Any involvement with the medical system increases parents' and children's knowledge. Those involved over long periods of time become masters at working the system effectively. Often, they become advocates for friends or relatives who call for advice or support. They are no longer intimidated by the hospital, they understand why and how things work, and they use this knowledge to help others.

- **Knowledge about illness and injuries.** Both children and parents learn a great deal about illness, death and dying, kindness, and ways to help people who are hurting. They develop a true compassion from their experiences in the hospital and the friends they made there. Many children who have endured long hospitalizations, as well as their siblings, plan careers in the helping professions. It can transform their lives.

- **Confidence.** The confidence of "having been there, done that" hones children's and parents' abilities to help others in crisis. They know just the right things to say and do when a friend is in the hospital. They are comfortable visiting the hospital, talking to doctors, offering help, and sending caring letters. Their medical competence is high.

Best wishes for a positive hospital experience for you, your child, and your entire family. May your child be well-prepared, warmly treated, healed of the illness or injury, and home soon.

# My Hospital Journal

*My name:*_____

_____

_____

*Date I came to the hospital:*_____

_____

_____

*Name of the hospital:*_____

_____

_____

# Before I came
# to the hospital

*What I thought it would be like:*_____

_____

_____

_____

_____

*What my parents told me:*_____

_____

_____

_____

*The hospital tour:*_____

_____

_____

*What I packed:*_____

_____

_____

_____

_____

# My room

*My room number:*_____

*My bed:*_____

*What I see out my window:*_____

_____

_____

_____

_____

_____

*How I decorate my room:* _____

_____

_____

_____

_____

_____

_____

_____

_____

_____

# Why I am
# in the hospital

*How my parents describe it:*_____

_____

_____

_____

_____

*How my doctor describes it:*_____

_____

_____

_____

_____

*What I think of it:*_____

_____

_____

_____

_____

_____

# My doctor(s)

My doctor's name:_____

_____

What I call him:_____

_____

_____

What I like best about my doctor:_____

_____

_____

Something I don't like:_____

_____

_____

My doctor writes a note:_____

_____

_____

_____

_____

_____

# My nurses

*My nurses' names:*_____

_____

_____

*What I call them:*_____

_____

_____

*What I like best about my nurses:*_____

_____

_____

*Something I don't like:*_____

_____

_____

*My nurses write a note:*_____

_____

_____

_____

_____

_____

# My roommate(s)

*My roommate's name:*_____

_____

_____

*Why my roommate is in the hospital:*_____

_____

_____

*Where my roommate lives:*_____

_____

_____

*What I like about sharing a room:*_____

_____

_____

*What I don't like:*_____

_____

_____

_____

_____

_____

# My school

*My teacher's name:*_____

_____

_____

*My best friends at school:*_____

_____

*My favorite subject:*_____

_____

_____

*How my class will know I'm in the hospital:*_____

_____

_____

*How many days of school I am missing:*_____

_____

_____

*How I do my homework:*_____

_____

_____

_____

# People who send me cards or gifts

_____

_____

_____

_____

_____

_____

_____

_____

_____

_____

_____

_____

_____

_____

_____

_____

# Friends' sign-in sheet

# Relatives' sign-in sheet

# Meals in the hospital

What I order for meals:_____
_____
_____

Favorite breakfast:_____

Favorite lunch:_____

Favorite dinner:_____

Hospital food I don't like:_____
_____

How eating in the hospital is different from eating at home:_____
_____

Food I can't have:_____
_____

# Other places I've been to in the hospital

__ *Lobby*

__ *Gift shop*

__ *Cafeteria*

__ *Playroom*

__ *Elevator*

__ *Operating room*

__ *Recovery room*

__ *Nurses' station*

__ *X-ray room*

*Others:*_____

_____

_____

_____

_____

_____

_____

# What happens at night in the hospital

What it sounds like:_____

_____

_____

_____

When the nurses come in:_____

_____

_____

_____

What nurses do at night:_____

_____

_____

_____

What I like:_____

_____

_____

What I don't like:_____

_____

# What I miss from home

*My brother(s):*_____

_____

_____

*My sister(s):*_____

_____

_____

*My pets:*_____

_____

*My friends:*_____

_____

*My bed:*_____

_____

_____

*What else?*_____

_____

_____

_____

_____

# Playing in the hospital

How I play in my room:_____

_____

_____

What the hospital playroom is like:_____

_____

_____

How I go to the playroom:_____

_____

_____

Who helps kids in the playroom:_____

_____

_____

What toys are there:_____

_____

_____

Other kids I met in the playroom:_____

_____

_____

# Medicine

Pills I have to take:_____

_____

_____

How the pills taste:_____

_____

_____

Liquid medicine I have to take:_____

_____

_____

How that tastes:_____

_____

_____

How often I have medicine:_____

_____

Medicines I have to bring home with me:_____

_____

How I feel about my medicines:_____

_____

# Tests in the hospital

___ CAT scan

___ X-ray

___ Blood draw

*Others:*_____

_____

*Tests I like the best:*_____

_____

_____

_____

*Tests I don't like:*_____

_____

_____

_____

*Prizes I get:*_____

_____

_____

_____

# Operation

What my operation is for:_____

_____

_____

Where my scar is:_____

_____

What my bandages look like:_____

_____

_____

How long my operation took:_____

_____

My surgeon's name:_____

_____

What I remember:_____

_____

_____

_____

_____

_____

# Going home

The day I left the hospital:_____

_____

_____

How long I stayed:_____

_____

_____

How I felt about leaving:_____

_____

_____

Who drove me home:_____

_____

_____

How I went from my room to the front door:_____

_____

_____

What it was like outside:_____

_____

_____

# Memories

*What I remember most:*_____

_____

_____

_____

_____

_____

_____

_____

*How I'll feel if I have to go to the hospital again:*

_____

_____

_____

_____

_____

_____

_____

# Packing List

## Clothing
____ shirts

____ pants

____ underwear

____ pajamas

____ bathrobe

____ slippers

____ shoes

____ socks

## For the room
____ blankets

____ bedspread/quilt

____ comfy pillow

____ clock

____ pictures of family, friends, pets

____ posters

____ tape to put up pictures and posters

____ balloons/streamers/ crepe paper

____ books for parents

____ magazines

____ stationery and stamps

____ address book

____ snack foods and drinks

## Toys
____ stuffed animals

____ dolls

____ children's books

____ playing cards

____ board games

____ puzzles

____ puppets

____ craft projects

____ video tapes

____ tape player or CD boom box

____ audio tapes or CDs

____ squirt gun

____ pens, pencils, paper

____ art materials: markers, paints, crayons

## Hygiene
____ eyeglasses

____ toothbrush

____ toothpaste

____ dental floss

153

___ tissues

___ body lotion

___ powder

___ shampoo/conditioner

___ soap

___ brush/comb

___ nail clippers

___ earplugs

## Miscellaneous

___ food

___ camera and film

___ money

___ sewing kit

___ safety pins

___ hot water bottle

___ flashlight

# Resources

## Books for young children

Ciliotta, Claire, and Carole Livingston. *Why am I Going to the Hospital?* Secaucus, NJ: Lyle Stuart Inc., 1981.

Hautzig, Deborah. *A Visit to the Sesame Street Hospital.* New York: Random House, 1985.

Rey, Margaret, and H. A. Rey. *Curious George Goes to the Hospital.* New York: Houghton Mifflin, 1966.

Rockwell, Anne, and Harlow Rockwell. *The Emergency Room.* New York: MacMillan, 1985.

Rogers, Fred. *Going to the Hospital.* New York: G.P. Putnam's & Sons, 1988.

## Books for older children

Howe, James. *The Hospital Book.* New York: Crown Publishers, 1981.

Richter, Elizabeth. *The Teenage Hospital Experience: You Can Handle It.* New York: Coward, McCann, and Geohegan, 1982.

## Books for siblings

Duncan, Debbie. *When Molly Was in the Hospital: A Book for Brothers and Sisters of Hospitalized Children.* Minimed series, Volume 1. Windsor, CA: Rayve Productions, 1994.

Allan Peterkin. *What About Me? When Brothers and Sisters Get Sick*. Washington, DC: Magination, 1992.

# Books and videos for parents

Child Life Council. *Preparing Your Child for Repeated or Extended Hospitalizations*. Available from: 11820 Parklawn Drive #202, Rockville, MD, 20852. (301) 881-7090. $11.50.

Johnson, Joy. *Why Mine? A Book for Parents Whose Child is Seriously Ill*. Omaha, NE: Centering Corporation, 1981. To order, call (402) 553-1200.

Keene, Nancy. *Working with Your Doctor: Getting the Healthcare You Deserve*. Sebastopol, CA: O'Reilly & Associates, Inc., 1998.

Kuttner, Leora, Ph.D. *A Child In Pain: How to Help, What to Do*. Point Roberts, WA: Hartley & Marks, 1996.

Kuttner, Leora, Ph.D. *No Fears, No Tears*. Videotape. Available through the Canadian Cancer Society: 265 West Tenth Avenue, Vancouver, BC, V5Z 4J4, Canada. Phone: (604) 872-4400; *http://www.bc.cancer.ca/ccs/*.

Kuttner, Leora, Ph.D. *No Fears, No Tears—13 Years Later*. Videotape. To order, fax your request to: (604) 294-9986, or send email to: *leora_kuttner@sfu.ca*.

Lewis, Sheldon, and Sheila Lewis. *Stress Proofing Your Child: Mind-Body Exercises to Enhance Your Child's Health*. New York: Bantam Books, 1996.

National Information Center for Children and Youth With Disabilities. *Meeting the Medical Bills*. To order, call 1 (800) 695-0285.

O'Connell, Avice, and Norma Leone. *Your Child and X-Rays: A Parents' Guide to Radiation and Other Imaging Procedures*. Rochester, NY: Lion Press, 1988.

Peterson, Sheila. *A Special Way to Care.* 1988. Available from: Friends of Karen, Box 217, Croton Falls, NY, 10519.

# Helpful organizations

Association for the Care of Children's Health
19 Mantua Road
Mt. Royal, NJ 08061
(609) 224-1742
Fax: (609) 423-3420
Email: *amkent@smarthub.com*
*http://ww.acch.org/acch*

Helps families of hospitalized children. Call to get their free resource list containing dozens of helpful books, brochures, and videotapes on preparing for health care experiences, pain and relaxation resources, pediatric AIDS, premature babies, and many other topics related to children's hospitalizations.

## Places to stay near hospitals

National Association of Hospital Hospitality Houses
1 (800) 542-9730

Provides referrals to free or low-cost lodging near medical facilities.

Ronald McDonald Houses
c/o Golin/Harris Communications, Inc.
111 East Wacker Drive, 10th Floor
Chicago, IL 60614
(312) 729-4000

Provides free or low-cost housing close to hospitals in many major cities for ill children and their families.

# Free air travel

National Patient Air Transport Helpline
1 (800) 296-1217 (United States)
(757) 318-9145 (elsewhere)
Email: *npathmsg@aol. com*
*http://www.npath.org*

Information and referral for free or discount air travel for patients who must travel to a distant location for specialized treatment or recovery after an illness or injury.

# Help with finances

Patient Advocate Foundation
739 Thimble Shoals Blvd., Suite 704
Newport News, VA 23606
(757) 873-6668
Fax: (757) 873-8999
Email: *PAF@acor.org*
*http://www.medinfo.org.* Click on "Organizations."

Provides information on managed care/insurance issues, legal counseling about financial debt intervention, and insurance denials of coverage.

# Free medical care

St. Jude Children's Research Hospital
332 North Lauderdale Street
Memphis, TN 38101
(901) 495-3300

Treats over 4,000 children yearly for catastrophic childhood illnesses including cancer, acquired and inherited immunodeficiencies, and genetic disorders. St. Jude was founded by Danny Thomas in 1962, and is funded by The American Lebanese Syrian Associated Charities (ALSAC). All costs of care beyond those reimbursable by third party payments are covered (including transportation and local living expenses).

Shriner's Hospitals for Children
PO Box 31356
Tampa, FL 33631
1 (800) 237-5055 (United States)
1 (800) 361-7256 (Canada)
*http:// www.shrinershq. org*

Twenty-two hospitals that provide expert free medical care for children with orthopedic problems and burn-related conditions.

## Stress reduction

The Academy for Guided Imagery
PO Box 2070
Mill Valley, CA 94942
1 (800) 726-2070

A professional organization that will direct you to a practitioner in your area who is skilled in teaching children visualization techniques.

The American Society of Clinical Hypnosis
2200 East Devon Avenue, Suite 291
Des Plaines, IL 60018
(847) 297-3317
*http://www.asch.net*

A professional organization of doctors, Ph.D. psychologists, and dentists that will refer you to local members on request. Send a stamped, self-addressed envelope.

Starbright Foundation
1990 South Bundy Drive, Suite 100
Los Angeles, CA 90025
(310) 442-1560
Fax: (310) 442-1568
*http://www.starbright.org*

Co-chaired by Steven Spielberg and Gen. Norman Schwarzkopf, Starbright Foundation creates products and programs for kids and teens with serious illness. It is best known for its online network of interactive, virtual-reality playgrounds where hospitalized children across the country meet, talk, and play. Such meetings help children cope with the pain, stress, and anxiety caused by medical treatments.

Starbright's "Videos With Attitude" help teens understand what its like to be ill, and frequently hospitalized, by listening to kids who have "been there, done that." For example, *What am I, Chopped Liver? Communicating with your Doctor* teaches how to speak up, ask questions, and feel more in control. The videos are free to families and come with a parent guide.

# Contributors

Brenda Andrews, L. S. Auth, Jodie Barbour, Robin B., Sue Brooks, Edie Cardwell, Carolyn J. Casey, Alicia Cauley, Wendy Corder Dowhower, Debra Ethier, S. Farringer, Lisa Hall, Connie Higbee-Jones, Chris Hurley, Missy Layfield, Deirdre McCarthy-King, Sara McDonnall, Wendy Mitchell, Amanda Moodie, Ann and Mark Newman, Robin Aspman-O'Callahan, Tim and Christina O'Reilly, Carrie Beth Parigrew, M. Clare Paris, Sandra L. Pilant, Mary C. Riecke, Jennifer M. Rohloff, Sheila Sandiford, Carol Schuette, Brenna Scoville, Scott and Richelle Shields, Cathi Poer Smith, Carl and Diane Snedeker, Ralene Walls, Emily Weiner, Kimbra Suzanne Wilder, Jean Wilkinson, Ellen Zimmerman.

# About the Authors

Nancy Keene lives in Washington state and is busy writing and raising two daughters. She has been involved with the medical world for over two decades. She has worked as both a paramedic and emergency medical technician (EMT) instructor. She also spent many years advocating for and supporting her young daughter through intensive treatment for acute leukemia.

Nancy's first book, *Childhood Leukemia: A Guide for Families, Friends, and Caregivers*, blends technical information with stories from over forty parents, children with cancer, and their siblings. She is also the author of *Working with Your Doctor: Getting the Healthcare You Deserve*, published in 1998, and co-author of *Childhood Cancer Survivors: A Guide to the Future,* to be published in fall 1999. Nancy spends considerable time talking with parents of children newly diagnosed with cancer, and is a tireless defender of children's medical rights.

Rachel Prentice is a graduate student at the Massachusetts Institute of Technology. She worked for eight years as a newspaper reporter in Washington state, New Mexico, and Rome, Italy. She has extensive experience writing about science, technology, and the environment. She has won acclaim and awards for newspaper articles on a wide range of topics.

# Colophon

Patient-Centered Guides are about the experience of illness. They contain personal stories as well as a mixture of practical and medical information.

The faces on the covers of our Guides reflect the human side of the information we offer.

The cover of *Your Child in the Hospital: A Practical Guide for Parents, Second Edition,* was designed by Edie Freedman and implemented by Kathleen Wilson, using Adobe Photoshop 5.0 and QuarkXPress 3.32. The cover photo is Copyright © 1994 by Hank Morgan, and is used with permission.

The interior layout of this book was designed by Edie Freedman and implemented by Kathleen Wilson, using QuarkXPress 3.32. The fonts used are Onyx BT and Berkeley from the Bitstream Foundry.

This book was proofread by Kimberly Brown. Mary Anne Weeks Mayo, Claire Cloutier LeBlanc, John Files, and Sheryl Avruch conducted quality control checks.

# Patient-Centered Guides™

## Questions Answered
## Experiences Shared

*We are committed to empowering individuals to evolve
into informed consumers armed with the latest information and
heartfelt support for their journey.*

When your life is turned upside down, your need for information is great. You have to make critical medical decisions, often with what seems little to go on. Plus you have to break the news to family, quiet your own fears, cope with symptoms or treatment side effects, figure out how you're going to pay for things, and sometimes still get to work or get dinner on the table.

*Patient-Centered Guides* provide authoritative information for intelligent information seekers who want to become advocates of their own health. They cover the whole impact of illness on your life. In each book, there's a mix of:

- **Medical background for treatment decisions**
  We can give you information that can help you to intelligently work with your doctor to come to a decision. We start from the viewpoint that modern medicine has much to offer and also discuss complementary treatments. Where there are treatment controversies we present differing points of view.

- **Practical information**
  Once you've decided what to do about your illness, you still have to deal with treatments and changes to your life. We cover day-to-day practicalities, such as those you'd hear from a good nurse or a knowledgeable support group.

- **Emotional support**
  It's normal to have strong reactions to a condition that threatens your life or changes how you live. It's normal that the whole family is affected. We cover issues like the shock of diagnosis, living with uncertainty, and communicating with loved ones.

Each book also contains stories from both patients and doctors—medical "frequent fliers" who share, in their own words, the lessons and strategies they have learned when maneuvering through the often complicated maze of medical information that's available.

We provide information online, including updated listings of the resources that appear in this book. This is freely available for you to print out and copy to share with others, as long as you retain the copyright notice on the print-outs.

## *http://www.patientcenters.com*

# Other Books in the Series

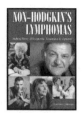

## Non-Hodgkin's Lymphomas
### Making Sense of Diagnosis, Treatment, and Options
By Lorraine Johnston
ISBN 1-56592-444-4, Paperback, 6" x 9", 535 pages, $24.95

*This complete guide helps those living with non-Hodgkin's lymphomas (NHL) to participate in wise treatment decisions. Topics include current treatment options, clinical trials, coping with tests, symptoms, and treatment side effects, communicating with medical personnel, and handling insurance and finances.*

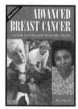

## Advanced Breast Cancer
### A Guide to Living with Metastatic Disease, 2nd Edition
By Musa Mayer
ISBN 1-56592-522-X, Paperback, 6" x 9", 536 pages, $19.95

*"An excellent book...if knowledge is power, this book will be good medicine."*

—David Spiegel, MD
Stanford University
Author of *Living Beyond Limits*

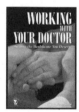

## Working with Your Doctor
### Getting the Healthcare You Deserve
By Nancy Keene
ISBN 1-56592-273-5, Paperback, 6" x 9", 380 pages, $15.95

*"Working with Your Doctor fills a genuine need for patients and their family members caught up in this new and intimidating age of impersonal, economically driven health care delivery. Upon finishing this eminently readable book, the only question left unanswered is why Nancy Keene didn't give it to us sooner. Patients and doctors alike owe her a large debt of gratitude."*

—James Dougherty, MD
Emeritus Professor of Surgery
Albany Medical College

***Patient-Centered Guides***
Published by O'Reilly & Associates, Inc.
Our products are available at a bookstore near you.
For information: **800-998-9938** • **707-829-0515** • **info@oreilly.com**
101 Morris Street • Sebastopol • CA • 95472-9902

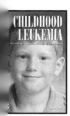

## Childhood Leukemia
### A Guide for Families, Friends & Caregivers
By Nancy Keene
ISBN 1-56592-191-7, Paperback, 6" x 9", 566 pages, $24.95

*"What's so compelling about Childhood Leukemia is the amount of useful medical information and practical advice it contains. A valuable resource to help parents and children regain their equilibrium after diagnosis and during the next two to three years of treatment, it answers questions requiring immediate attention. Keene avoids jargon and lays out what's needed to deal with the medical system."*

—The Washington Post

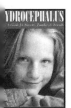

## Hydrocephalus
### A Guide for Patients, Families & Friends
By Chuck Toporek and Kellie Robinson
ISBN 1-56592-410-X, Paperback, 6" x 9", 382 pages, $19.95

*"In this book, the authors have provided a wonderful entry into the world of hydrocephalus to begin to remedy the neglect of this important condition. We are immensely grateful to them for their groudbreaking effort."*

—Peter D. Black, M.D., Ph.D.
Franc D. Ingraham Professor of Neurosurgery,
Harvard Medical School
Neurosurgeon in Chief,
Brigham and Women's Hospital,
Children's Hospital
Boston, Massachusetts

## Choosing a Wheelchair
### A Guide for Optimal Independence
By Gary Karp
ISBN 1-56592-411-8, Paperback, 5" x 8", 190 pages, $9.95

*"I love the idea of putting knowledge often possessed only by professionals into the hands of new consumers. Gary Karp has done it. This book will empower people with disabilities to make informed equipment choices."*

—Barry Corbet, Editor
New Mobility Magazine

### Patient-Centered Guides
*Published by O'Reilly & Associates, Inc.*
Our products are available at a bookstore near you.
For information: **800-998-9938** • **707-829-0515** • info@oreilly.com
101 Morris Street • Sebastopol • CA • 95472-9902